STAGING WOMEN AND
THE SOUL-BODY DYNAMIC
IN EARLY MODERN ENGLAND

Women and Gender in the Early Modern World

Series Editors:
Allyson Poska, The University of Mary Washington, USA
Abby Zanger

The study of women and gender offers some of the most vital and innovative challenges to current scholarship on the early modern period. For more than a decade now, Women and Gender in the Early Modern World has served as a forum for presenting fresh ideas and original approaches to the field. Interdisciplinary and multidisciplinary in scope, this Ashgate book series strives to reach beyond geographical limitations to explore the experiences of early modern women and the nature of gender in Europe, the Americas, Asia, and Africa. We welcome proposals for both single-author volumes and edited collections which expand and develop this continually evolving field of study.

Titles in the series

Masculinity and Marian Efficacy in Shakespeare's England
Ruben Espinosa

Reading the Jewish Woman on the Elizabethan Stage
Michelle Ephraim

Midwiving Subjects in Shakespeare's England
Caroline Bicks

Beard Fetish in Early Modern England
Sex, Gender, and Registers of Value
Mark Albert Johnston

Biblical Women's Voices in Early Modern England
Michele Osherow

English Women, Religion, and Textual Production, 1500–1625
Edited by Micheline White

Printing and Parenting in Early Modern England
Edited by Douglas A. Brooks

Staging Women and
the Soul-Body Dynamic
in Early Modern England

SARAH E. JOHNSON
Queen's University, Canada

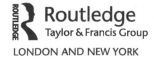

LONDON AND NEW YORK

First published 2014 by Ashgate Publishing

Published 2016 by Routledge
2 Park Square, Milton Park, Abingdon, Oxfordshire OX14 4RN
711 Third Avenue, New York, NY 10017, USA

First issued in paperback 2016

Routledge is an imprint of the Taylor & Francis Group, an informa business

British Library Cataloguing in Publication Data
A catalogue record for this book is available from the British Library

The Library of Congress has cataloged the printed edition as follows:
Johnson, Sarah E., author.
 Staging Women and the Soul-Body Dynamic in Early Modern England / by Sarah E. Johnson.
     pages cm.—(Women and Gender in the Early Modern World)
  Includes index.
  ISBN 978-1-4724-1122-8 (hardcover: alk. paper)—

  1. English drama—Early modern and Elizabethan, 1500–1600—History and criticism.
2. English drama—17th century—History and criticism. 3. Women in literature. 4. Women and literature—Great Britain—History—16th century. 5. Women and literature—Great Britain—History—17th century. I. Title.
  PR649.W66J64 2014
  822'.3093522—dc23

                                                                      2013035088

ISBN 13: 978-1-138-24847-2 (pbk)
ISBN 13: 978-1-4724-1122-8 (hbk)

For Arden

Contents

Acknowledgements

The first of my thanks to those who assisted me as I developed this study I owe to Helen Ostovich. I am deeply grateful for her supportive mentorship over the years and for her confidence in my work. I have also learned much from Helen's great talents as an editor and have found energy and elegance to emulate in her writing. Marta Straznicky generously fulfilled the role of postdoctoral supervisor, warmly welcomed me into the Queen's community, and engaged thoughtfully and encouragingly with my work. I have frequently counted on her discerning and excellent advice. Two of the graduate seminars that Mary Silcox taught during my time at McMaster planted the seeds for this book's topic and influenced my thinking about the importance of soul-body ideas in the period. I am appreciative, too, of comments Mary provided on previous versions of these chapters. I aspire to Melinda Gough's model of rigorous scholarship and I am indebted to her for insightful, thorough, and enthusiastic responses to this work in its earlier stages. Chapter 4, in particular, benefitted from discussion with Melinda. I wish to extend my thanks to Jennifer Panek for her careful reading of an early version of the manuscript and for her judicious comments and suggestions, as well as to Betty Ann Levy and Catherine Graham for their thought-provoking questions and good humour. Thank you also to Gabrielle Sugar, Deanna Smid, Johnathan Pope, and Jessica Dell for sharing their friendship over the course of this project and beyond.

I thank Erika Gaffney at Ashgate Publishing, who is a pleasure to work with, and Kirsten Giebutowski and Louise Watson for their careful treatment of the manuscript. This study also profited from the generous, constructive, and much appreciated feedback I received from its anonymous reader.

The Social Sciences and Humanities Research Council of Canada funded my doctoral and postdoctoral studies, which enabled me to begin this project and see it through to publication. A portion of Chapter 2 was published previously as '"A Spirit to Resist" and Female Eloquence in *The Tamer Tamed*', *Shakespeare* 7.3 (2011): 309–24, and is included in this study by permission of the publisher, Taylor & Francis Ltd, http://www.tandf.co.uk/journals. Material from Chapter 4 appeared as 'The Female Body as Soul in Queen Anna's Masques', and is reprinted with permission from *SEL Studies in English Literature 1500–1900* 53.2 (Spring 2013): 357–77.

Those whose love and support I have felt in every situation and endeavour also deserve thanks, of course, for their encouragement in this particular endeavour. I thank my parents, Darlene and Raymond Johnson, most of all. I thank my sisters, Krista and Laura, and I thank the Collins clan. I thank my dear friend Desirée Phillips for her kind words. And last only for emphasis, I acknowledge that this book is just one of many things that would not have been possible without the love, understanding, and help of the one I am so grateful to have as my partner, Tim Collins.

Note on Texts

I accessed all early books cited in this study through *Early English Books Online* (*EEBO*). I have preserved original spelling and have silently modernized letters (such as the long s, i/j, u/v) and expanded contractions.

All references to the *Oxford English Dictionary* are to the *OED* Online.

Introduction
Women and the Soul-Body Dynamic

Literary Convention, Literal Consequences

In early modern England, calling into question whether women possessed souls meant calling into question their intelligence, their capacity for reason, their ability to govern their own bodies and passions. It also meant departing from the orthodox Christian belief that men and women were both created in God's image, with an immaterial, immortal component to the self. And yet the idea that women might be soulless circulated as a theological proposition and as a form of academic joke. John Donne even played with this idea in one of his early writings.

The seventh Problem of Donne's *Paradoxes and Problems* is, as its title announces, '*Why hath the common opinion affoorded woemen Soules?*' To solve this riddle, Donne first elaborates on why attributing souls to women is questionable. First, 'wee' – the pronoun signalling a targeted male audience – do not even receive 'any part' of our 'mortall soules of sence or growth' from 'them'.[1] On top of this apparent learned consensus, 'wee dynye soules to others' who 'equall' women in 'all but Speeche', and after all, women owe their speech 'onely to theyr bodily instruments'. Who are these 'others' equal to women? Donne speculates that an ape, goat, fox, or serpent could speak just as well as a woman if they possessed the same mechanisms for speech. So why do men persist in accrediting women with souls? Maybe to avoid displeasing women, since they have 'so many' ways to 'hurt' men. 'Even theyr loving destroyes us', Donne points out. Men therefore 'give them what they will', and when some call women 'Angels' or 'Goddesses', and 'the Peputian Heretikes make them Bishops', men get carried away and 'allow them soules' too. Or perhaps men dignify women in this way only to 'flatter' those princes and 'great personages' who are 'so much governed' by women. Donne piles up these contemptuous examples. Maybe men say women have souls as a means of overlooking their own prodigality: if even a woman possesses a soul, a soul must be 'no greate matter' to concern oneself with. Yet again, men may simply 'lend' women souls for use, since women will give their souls away again, along with their bodies. These answers culminate in the final suggestion that men allow women souls since women 'would come neere' the devil, and the devil, 'who doth most mischeefe', is 'all soule'. In other words, perhaps to repay women for the miseries they cause, men 'have given woemen soules onely to make them capable of damnation'.

---

[1]   John Donne, 'Why Hath the Common Opinion Affoorded Woemen Soules?', 28–9. All subsequent quotations of this work come from these page numbers.

Donne is careful to prevent the uncontrolled circulation of early writings like this one, entreating Henry Goodyer in a letter to 'let goe no copy of my Problems, till I review them. If it be too late, at least be able to tell me who hath them'.[2] Helen Peters endorses Evelyn Simpson's suggestion that in order to avoid offending those who might help him rehabilitate his career, Donne likely revised certain Problems (namely, 'XVIII on "Women and Feathers"' and 'XII on the "Variety of Green"') that conveyed 'hostility' or 'bitterness' towards women or towards the court.[3] Despite Donne's apparent unease about who might chance to read his Paradoxes or Problems, literary critics of these works have emphasized that if we take their content at face value – if we dwell, for instance, on the blatant misogyny of Problem VII – we are missing the point. Instead, we should notice how Donne's Problems work to parody or criticize the very scholarly practice and literary form they exemplify. We should recognize that they encourage the careful reader to resist their showy rhetoric.[4] Donne himself even calls his Paradoxes, closely related to the Problems in literary form and tradition, mere 'swaggerers' that 'do there [sic] office' if 'they make you to find better reasons against them'.[5]

If we apply to Problem VII this reading of the *Paradoxes and Problems* as exposing the limitations or dangers of stylized rhetorical display, however, we risk brushing aside the fact that the Problem dealing with women's souls flaunts adept skill at the type of rhetorical exercise that it purportedly parodies. Very little in this particular Problem suggests that its main purpose is to warn the reader about the potentially misleading qualities of rhetoric by showing how easily it can be mobilized to develop wrong ideas, such as the doubtfulness of women possessing souls. Instead, in keeping with the classical and university traditions to which the Problem form belongs, the more obvious effect of Problem VII is to entertain the reader through its display of the writer's cleverness – a display that in this case takes place entirely at women's expense. Simpson traces the Problem as an educational tool from its classical origins to its use in early modern England. It was featured in university exercises and annual disputations, and in formal demonstrations of wit and argument when royalty or dignitaries came to visit. Donne's familiarity with the disputation and the Problem would have come from his studies at Oxford and perhaps Cambridge.[6] His letters show that he also participated in the Problem's development 'as a means of social diversion'.[7] Problem VII's male scholar perspective comes through in its firm 'wee' and 'them' division that defines men

---

[2]   John Donne, 'To Sir [Henry Goodyer]', 383–4.

[3]   Helen Peters (ed.), *Paradoxes and Problems*, xli–xlii. Peters, xv–xvi, dates the Problems between 1603 and 1609 or 1610, 'a gloomy time in Donne's life for he lived in Mitcham with a sickly wife and an increasing family, without any proper means of support'.

[4]   See, for instance, James Baumlin, *John Donne and the Rhetorics of Renaissance Discourse*, 16–17, 65, 242, and Peters, *Paradoxes and Problems*, xl.

[5]   John Donne, *Complete Poetry and Selected Prose*, 378.

[6]   Evelyn Simpson, *Prose Works of John Donne*, xxxi.

[7]   Ibid.

as thinking subjects and women as interpretable material, a division very much in line with the traditional gendering of the rational soul as masculine and the body as feminine. George Parfitt claims that 'as a category women are objects for Donne's wit and of interest only in that respect', and that the focus here is on 'male commonplaces' or 'characteristics men assign to women' and not on a 'real revaluation of Woman'.[8] This distinction between the serious conceptualization of women versus simply the use of women as topic for an exercise in wit is, I think, a false one that, along with the characterization of Donne's Problems as 'clever trifles' produced nonchalantly 'at odd moments in a busy life',[9] dismisses the real cultural impact that the literary circulation of such stereotypes could carry for real women.

The negative stereotypes packed into Problem VII include: women are primarily bodily creatures, akin to animals in their irrationality; the contrary association of women with non-physical figures like angels or goddesses is meaningless flattery; women are of consequence only in their relations to men; and women are prone to losing their souls and jeopardizing men's through their alacrity for bodily lust. As this study will seek to unfold, the treatment of women in much early modern writing, as in Donne's 'Why Hath the Common Opinion Affoorded Woemen Soules?', is inextricable from common understandings of the soul-body divide itself as gendered. I begin with Donne's Problem VII in part because it starts to illustrate how the conventional gendering of the soul-body relationship is at once debilitating and deeply problematic for women, and yet something that risks being overlooked as mere convention, as unimportant because it does not really reflect sincere belief. Surely Donne, the future esteemed dean of St Paul's, would never have seriously entertained the idea that only men possessed souls? And yet, if the speculation that Donne worried about a 'possible patroness' seeing some of his Problems and taking offence does not convince that they are something more than harmless 'trifles', Simpson draws our attention to a telling passage in one of Donne's later sermons that could almost be taken as Donne speaking directly to his younger, Problem-writing self:

> For, howsoever some men out of a petulancy and wantonnesse of wit, and out of the extravagancy of Paradoxes, and such singularities, have called the faculties, and abilities of women in question, even in the roote thereof, in the reasonable and immortall soul, yet that one thing alone [the questioning of whether women possess souls] hath been enough to create a doubt, (almost an assurance in the negative) whether S. *Ambroses* Commentaries upon the Epistles of S. *Paul*, be truly his or no. ... No author of gravity, of piety, of conversation in the Scriptures could admit that doubt, whether a woman were created in the Image of God, that is, in possession of a reasonable and immortall soul.[10]

---

[8] George A.E. Parfitt, *John Donne: A Literary Life*, 32.
[9] Simpson, *Prose Works of John Donne*, 132, 148.
[10] Ibid., 142.

If an early modern reader of a writing like Donne's Problem VII would inevitably view its misogynistic wit as unconnected to ideas about real women, and if few credited the historical notion that women were soulless, despite this notion's availability for use in rhetorical stances, Donne would not likely have needed to explicitly and publicly address – and firmly denounce – this position as he does here, in a sermon he gave on Easter, 1630. Even earnest rejections of the argument that women lacked souls somehow lend weight to the topic as legitimate and worth consideration to begin with. Regardless of how far Problem VII's cynicism is from Donne's personal belief about women and souls, the question about women's souls, as I discuss in Chapter 2, actually received serious attention in the sixteenth and seventeenth centuries.

Indeed, despite Robert Ray's characterization of Donne's Problems as 'usually pseudo-problems, false issues, and largely unexplainable', developed with 'the most outrageous, illogical, and unexpected "reasons" for the sake of entertainment',[11] Problem VII's development is not illogical or unexpected. In the first line Donne cites a consensus that men have not received 'so much from [women] as any part of eyther of our mortall soules of sence or growth' – that is, that not even the lower faculties of the soul (according to the inherited Aristotelian model) came from one's mother. Questions about the soul's origin – whether a child received a soul from the mother, father, from both parents, or directly from God – were certainly not settled in the early modern period as this first line would suggest. In a treatise published more than three decades after the writing of Donne's Problems, for instance, Henry Woolnor, in tackling the question of how one indivisible soul can emerge from two souls, admits that Aristotle's denial 'that females had any seede at all, being onely as the ground wherein seede is sowen' offers an easy answer, 'for then the soule proceeding from the soule of the father onely, there shall not need be two soules, nor one mingled of two'.[12] Woolner ends up rejecting Aristotle's position in favour of a less male-centred view of 'the spirituall seede of the soule' as something that is 'not in the severall seede of either sex ... but rather in both when but one' – as something that only comes to exist, in other words, when the souls of two parents 'cleave together ... at the instant of conception'.[13] Around the same time, however, William Harvey's influential medical writings countered this version of generation. As Eve Keller has shown, Harvey credited male semen exclusively as the 'spark of life' and represented it as possessing 'divinity' in contrast to the female, who served merely as a passive 'incubator' for the foetus.[14] This debate into the 1640s about whether or not women shared with men the role of communicating a soul to their offspring indicates how Donne's academic joke is not detached from real questions and concerns that had serious repercussions for cultural perceptions of women.

---

[11]   Robert H. Ray, *John Donne Companion*, 191.

[12]   Henry Woolnor, *True Originall of the Soule*, 110–11. Page numbers should be 210–11, but the page number after 208 reads 109, and the subsequent pages count from 109.

[13]   Ibid., 111–13.

[14]   Eve Keller, *Generating Bodies and Gendered Selves*, 112–19.

In other words, separating the soul-body dynamic as a literary convention or motif from more literal considerations of this relationship would amount to a false distinction, I think, akin to attempting to distinguish between the use of 'women' as a topic or prop for rhetorical exercise and genuine attitudes towards women. In the following chapters, then, I work from the premise that literary and dramatic representations of women were deeply connected to the possibilities that real women could see for themselves and to the cultural attitudes they faced on a daily basis. This study is, nonetheless, literary in focus and concentrates on dramatic treatments of the soul-body dynamic as it underlies and inflects representations of women. I do not attempt to chronicle evidence of how real women might have received and responded to the texts I examine, nor do I survey or analyze the vast and complex corpus of early modern philosophical, theological, devotional, and anatomical[15] writings on the soul-body relationship, although an awareness of these discourses necessarily informs my readings of the plays and masques that I consider. This study is more concerned with how the pervasive early modern mode of gendering and hierarchizing the soul in relation to the body is at the heart of many negative or disempowering representations of women and justifications of women's supposedly inherent inferiority to men. But if the conventional gendering of the soul-body hierarchy served as a patriarchal tool for women's subordination (as it explicitly did), it carries equal potential to promote empowering ideas of women. Precisely because of its pervasiveness, its familiarity, this in many ways oppressive construct, I argue, also provides an effective tool for reconceptualizations of gender relations, in that variations on the dominant version of the body-soul relationship would be recognizable and loaded with meaning in their departure from the well-known standard. This book aims to demonstrate how a critical sensitivity to the full complexity of a dramatic text's engagement with understandings of the soul-body, or immaterial-material dynamic can suggest new, and often more flexible and positive, readings of its representations of women – readings available to early modern audiences that we should not overlook.

A Word on Terms

Throughout this study I use the terms 'soul', 'spirit', 'mind', 'intellect', 'reason', and 'immaterial' somewhat interchangeably, as with the opposing terms 'body', 'flesh', 'matter', and 'material'. These terms indeed overlap and were often conflated in the language of early modern writers. So, while we must be aware of how 'spirit' could designate a specific kind of bridge between body and soul, 'a subtle and thin body always movable, engendered of blood and vapour, and the

---

[15] Johnathan Pope, 'Anatomy of the Soul', has exposed a lack of critical attention to how early modern anatomical works were concerned with the soul as well as with the body and contributed to, or reflected, the shaping of early modern subjectivity, as unstable and elusive as that subjectivity is to define.

vehicle or carriage of the faculties of the soul',[16] my usage reflects how, alongside this definition, 'spirit' could also simply be another word for 'soul'. John Davies's long poem *Nosce Teipsum* (1599), for example, claims that '*The Soul a Substance and a Spirit* is', a '*spirit* ... / Which from the fountaine of Gods spirit doth flow', and which is 'not like *aire* or *wind*, / Nor like the *spirits* about the *heart* or *braine*' (i.e., the 'spirits' of physiological discourse).[17] Davies also calls the soul 'a *spirit* and *immateriall mind*'.[18] Simon Harward's *Discourse Concerning the Soule and Spirit of Man* (1604) opens Chapter 1 with the subheading '*How many wayes the words Soule and Spirit are synonyma*' and proceeds to give several examples, including that both words 'point out' the intellect, that is, the 'rationall soul and understanding spirit'.[19] Some scholars warn that the opposition between spirit and flesh, however, is not always the same as the opposition between soul and body, primarily with reference to the Pauline tension between spirit and flesh as a tension between two different spiritual orientations, the way of the spirit leading towards God and the way of the flesh leading away from God.[20] The Platonic, Augustinian, and Aristotelian divisions of the soul into higher and lower faculties, however,

---

[16]   Helkiah Crooke, *Mikrokosmographia*, 3.12.173. William Hill, *Infancie of the Soule*, C3r, cites Hippocrates in his definition of 'Spirit' as the chair and instrument of the soul, noting that the Spirit, taking the forms of vital or lively spirit in the heart, natural spirit in the liver, and animal spirit in the head, joins together body and soul, and when the spirit is weak, the body-soul connection weakens. Gail Kern Paster, 'Nervous Tension', 113, 121, provides a critical assessment of the treatment of 'spirit' in physiological discourse, focusing on Helkiah Crooke. 'As properties animating, even defining the living body', spirits, she points out, 'like soul, eluded the anatomist; but, unlike soul, they mattered to his work because they were thought responsible for some of the body's most important structures of visible and behavioural difference, inside and out'. Paster's exploration of the physiological understanding of spirits leads her to posit that the discourse surrounding spirits 'provides a historically specific rationale for strong, ethically loaded contrasts between paired traits like impulsiveness versus self-containment, spontaneity versus calculation or strategic thinking'.

[17]   John Davies, *Nosce Teipsum*, C2v, D3v.

[18]   Ibid., E1r.

[19]   Simon Harward, *Discourse Concerning the Soule*, B1r, B4r. Harward, 8, also gives an account of the relationship between animal spirits and the soul, with an analogy cited as Galenic that the 'spirit is in respect of the soule, as the sparkle in respect of the fire'. He provides a lucid summary of how the three types of spirits – animal, vital, and natural – served by sinews, arteries, and veins, respectively, correspond to Plato's three faculties of the soul: Rational, Irascible, and Appetitory (9). For further examples of the slippage between 'soul' and 'spirit' or 'soul' and 'mind', see Nicholas Breton's *Solemne Passion of the Soules Love*, A2r; Woolnor's *True Originall of the Soule*, 13; John Woolton's *Immortalitie of the Soule*, fol. 14; and Thomas Wright's *Passions of the Minde*, 297, 300–301, in which he cites 'blindnesse of the Minde' as a proof of the imperfection of the soul, and, in a list of 'Problemes concerning the substance of our Soules', uses 'Spirit' in the sense of 'soul', and 'spirits' to refer to bodily substances, within the space of a few lines.

[20]   See, for instance, Kate Narveson, 'Flesh, Excrement, Humors, Nothing', 315–16, and Rosalie Osmond, *Mutual Accusation*, 10, 21, 35.

corresponded with the values attached to the larger division between soul and body and thus facilitated the conflation of these parallel dichotomies. My position is that, in the same way, the use of 'spirit' and 'flesh' as metaphorical vehicles for positive and negative spiritual orientations cannot be finally isolated from thinking about the actual soul and body.

Soul over Body, A Gendered Hierarchy

My designation thus far of the soul-body 'hierarchy' and my references to the most 'pervasive' or 'predominant' cultural coding of this relationship as gendered are not meant to belie the reality that early modern discourses concerning the body and soul are richly varied and complex, and even sometimes abandon altogether the prevalent model of this relationship as dichotomous. Nonetheless, when gender comes into play, as it so frequently does, the designation of the body as feminine and of the soul as masculine, in relation to each other, predominates, along with the assignment of certain key characteristics to each. Scholars such as Rosalie Osmond, Genevieve Lloyd, Thomas Laqueur, Ian Maclean, and W. Norris Clarke have already mapped the complex developments of body and soul theories from Plato (and earlier) into the early modern period, often with helpful attention to how these theories come to integrate gender.[21] I do not aim to recapitulate or revise

---

[21]   Thomas Laqueur, *Making Sex*, uses the term 'one-sex body' to refer to the historical understanding of man as the standard against which woman was defined, often as a flawed or lacking version of man. Laqueur explores how bodies have been understood as functioning differently in reproduction, not because of biological evidence, but because of cultural and philosophical beliefs about the nature of femininity and masculinity. Laqueur is an excellent source for nuanced explanations of the views of Aristotle, Hippocrates, and Galen – so influential in the Renaissance – on all aspects of generation. Historically, physiological and anatomical descriptions of the body, Laqueur argues, *had* to express women's inferiority, an inferiority that was culturally and politically pre-established. Ian Maclean, 'Notion of Woman', 135–6, see also 143–7, offers a comprehensive account of explanations in 'medicine, anatomy, and physiology' of women's constitution, especially those inherited from Aristotle and Galen, that contributed to the idea of woman as an imperfect or lesser version of man. 'Even after the abandonment of the "imperfect male" theory' (when, after 1580, the indication in most 'ancient texts' that 'woman is colder and moister in dominant humours' begins to be thought of as 'functional' instead of as a 'sign of imperfection'), Maclean finds that 'physiologists retain the beliefs in the less perfect mental faculties of woman'. See also Kate Aughterson (ed.), *Renaissance Woman: A Sourcebook*, 43. Sara Mendelson and Patricia Crawford, *Women in Early Modern England*, give a lucid account in the section on 'Medical Understandings of Woman's Body' of how 'medical and popular theories of the body ... constructed women's bodies as possessing dangerously unstable qualities. ... All assumed that women, unlike men, were created not as something in themselves, but rather for gestation and man's bodily convenience' (18–30). Norris W. Clarke, 'Living on the Edge', 183–99, traces the idea, from Plato into the Enlightenment, of the human as 'frontier being' straddling the dimensions of matter and spirit, with attention to the layering of Christian thought over the Platonic and Neoplatonic traditions.

this important work, but to build on it, turning what we know about concepts of body and soul in early modern England to new use in literary criticism. In order to explain my frequent recourse to the 'prevalent' or 'familiar' conceptualization of the soul-body relationship as gendered and hierarchical, however, a very brief review of some of this scholarship is necessary here.

The topic of the body-soul relationship received intense focus in early modern England. In *The Passions of the Minde* (1604) Thomas Wright gives an idea of this preoccupation in his complaint about the failure to achieve clarity on the subject:

> at least they [men] might have knowne themselves; for what was more neere them then their owne soules and bodies ... Yet the Ignorance and Errours, which both inchaunted them, and inveigle us, are almost incredible. I could propound above a hundreth questions about the Soule and the body, which partly are disputed of by Divines, partly by naturall and morall Philosophers, partly by Physitians, all which, I am of opinion, are so abstruse and hidden, that they might be defended as Problemes, and eyther parte of Contradiction alike impugned.[22]

William Hill conveys a similar sense of having to sort through a copious amount of material from a variety of disciplines in order to discuss *The Infancie of the Soule* (1605). He lists in his table of contents sections on poets', philosophers', physicians', and fathers' positions on the soul, as well as canonical and scriptural positions. Despite the wealth of material on the topic, recurring ideas do emerge. Scholars often identify the two most influential strands of thinking on this vital soul-body relationship in early modern England as deriving from Plato and Aristotle,[23] with due recognition that not every writer fits neatly into one or the other camp, and that further confusion arises from the frequent practice of 'uncritical' borrowing of 'snippets from different writers with contradictory opinions'.[24] Both Platonic and Aristotelian schools of thought hierarchize the components of soul and body in a way that corresponds and contributes to early modern notions of gender hierarchy. Plato separates the soul into the frequently cited three faculties of reason, will, and appetite (or the rational, spirited, and appetitive elements), located in the head, heart, and stomach, respectively. Osmond draws attention to the striking imagery Plato uses to privilege reason and separate it from the other faculties. In the *Timaeus*, 'the neck, which separates the rational faculty from the rest, Plato compares to an isthmus isolating it from contamination'.[25] Similarly,

---

[22]   Wright, *Passions of the Minde*, 300.

[23]   For a more in-depth explanation of Plato's and Aristotle's different takes on the soul-body relationship than I have space to offer here, and a full account of how Platonic and Aristotelian strains of thought came to early modern thinkers both directly and filtered through other philosophers, such as the Stoics, Plotinus, St Paul, Tertullian, Origen, Augustine, Aquinas, etc., refer to Osmond, *Mutual Accusation*, 7–17, and to Genevieve Lloyd, *Man of Reason*, 8, 19–37.

[24]   Osmond, *Mutual Accusation*, 22.

[25]   Ibid., 5.

in the *Phaedrus*'s famous chariot-and-horse analogy, the charioteer represents the 'rational faculty of the soul' directing 'the spirited element or will' (a white horse), which is a 'natural ally of reason', and 'the appetitive element' (the dark horse), which is prone to falling and tripping up the ensemble. Plato again isolates reason from the other faculties by figuring it entirely differently as a human figure and not as a lead horse.[26] He conceives of the soul as a hierarchy in which reason is at the top as the rightful governor of the other faculties, and hierarchy also structures his conception of the entire soul in relation to the body: 'Plato is clear that the imperfections we perceive, both on the individual and cosmic scale, come from the material, not the craftsman. It is the function of the soul to impose form on recalcitrant matter'.[27] Despite the fact that Plato's theories of body and soul were both complex and shifting, as they 'came to be selected by Christian philosophers, it was the dualistic elements that opposed a weak and fallible body to a soul with God-like affinities that predominated'.[28] To put it basically, the Platonic view in the Renaissance saw the soul as the rightful moral governor of a body that was an encumbrance to it, a prison, clog, or dunghill that the soul longed to escape.

At first Aristotle's emphasis on the body as necessary and good for the soul would seem to collapse Plato's hierarchy. While the senses are unreliable for Plato, for Aristotle they are 'our chief source of knowledge'.[29] Aristotle holds that 'neither body nor soul can be conceived of existing independently', and the 'intimacy' and 'functionality' of the body-soul relationship as he envisions it prevent a 'clear-cut, moral distinction' between the two of the kind that Plato describes.[30] Like Plato, however, Aristotle divides the soul and privileges rationality. In place of Plato's tripartite division, Aristotle imposes a binary separating the rational from the irrational soul. The irrational soul comprises the vegetative and sensitive faculties 'present in plant and animal life, so that nutrition, growth, and sense are all attributed to "soul"', while the rational soul separates into the active and passive intellect, with only the active intellect characterized by immortality.[31] Despite Aristotle's emphasis on the inextricable union of body and soul, his account of the intellect (*nous*), as Osmond records, was 'partly instrumental in reinforcing the passage of Platonic dualism into Christian thought'. A 'confusion between "mind" and "soul"' led later Christian philosophers to 'speak of the [entire] soul', and not

---

[26] Ibid.

[27] Ibid., 6.

[28] Ibid. Lloyd, *Man of Reason*, 7, also observes: 'In Plato's later thought, the simplicity of [the] subjection of body to mind gives way to a more complex location of the non-rational ... within the soul as a source of inner conflict. On this later view, the struggle is between a rational part of the soul and other non-rational parts that should be subordinated to it. Later Judaic and Christian thinkers elaborated this Platonic theme in ways that connected it explicitly with the theme of man's rightful domination of woman'.

[29] Osmond, *Mutual Accusation*, 6.

[30] Ibid., 6–7.

[31] Ibid., 7.

just a fragment of it, as at once 'naturally dependent on the body and yet retaining its qualities of immateriality and immortality'.[32] Besides this available use of Aristotle to support a dualistic conception of human nature, Aristotle's notion that the soul generates from male semen[33] lends support to a firm association of the soul with masculinity that held considerable sway in early modern England.

In claiming that women are physically incapable of producing seed to act as a vehicle for the soul in generation, and that the soul – along with that divine, active intellect – is passed down entirely through the father, Aristotle moves beyond the claim that women's bodies are inferior to men's. This bodily inferiority is an obstruction to complete affinity with the soul, an obstruction with which men do not have to contend. This idea stuck, and Genevieve Lloyd gives a brilliant account of it in her discussion of Augustine. Even while attempting to defend women as enjoying rational equality with men, Augustine cannot reject the notion of women as physically inferior to men nor escape the already deeply engrained cultural stereotypes of femininity that rest on the assertion of the weakness of female bodies. Augustine, Lloyd explains, tries to separate woman's subordinate position to man in terms of her bodily difference and her 'help-mate' role in Genesis from her status as an equally 'rational spirit':

> In respect of her rational intelligence, woman, like man, is subject to God alone. But her bodily difference from man, and the physical subjection which Augustine seems to see as inseparable from it, symbolically represents a subordination relation between two aspects of Reason. ... Woman's physical subordination to man symbolizes the rightful subordination of the mind's practical functions – its control over temporal things, managing the affairs of life – to its higher function in contemplating eternal things. The Genesis story of a helper for man having to be 'taken from himself and formed into his consort' symbolizes this diversion of Reason into practical [and lesser] affairs.

---

[32]   Ibid.

[33]   Osmond, *Mutual Accusation*, 7, n. 14, directs readers to a passage in Aristotle's *Generation of Animals* that explicitly designates male semen as the 'vehicle' for the soul. See also Laqueur, *Making Sex*, 29–30: with reference to Aristotle's claim that 'the female always provides the material, the male that which fashions it, for this is the power we say they each possess, and *this is what it means for them to be male and female* ... . While the body is from the female, it is the soul that is from the male', Laqueur comments that 'these were momentous distinctions, as powerful and plain as that between life and death. To Aristotle being male *meant* the capacity to supply the sensitive soul without which "it is impossible for face, hand, flesh, or any other part to exist" ... One sex was able to ... [produce] true sperma; the other was not'. For a helpful overview of Renaissance debate over 'female semen', how it compares to male semen (usually, it is 'less active'), and what it contributes to the foetus, see also Ian Maclean, *Renaissance Notion of Woman*, 35–7.

But, as Lloyd observes,

> despite [Augustine's] good intentions, his own symbolism pulls against his explicit doctrine of sexual equality with respect to the possession of Reason. ... [F]rom our perspective ... mere bodily difference surely makes the female no more appropriate than the male to the symbolic representation of 'lesser' intellectual functions. What is operating here ... is the conceptual alignment of maleness with superiority, femaleness with inferiority.[34]

In this glimpse of Augustine, we can see an easy, unquestioned correspondence between the hierarchy of the highest part of reason over its more practical functions (and more generally of eternal over mundane affairs and of soul over body), and a physical hierarchy of male over female – a correspondence that remained influential in early modern England. As with any analogy, however, this one works both ways.

Where Augustine claimed that men's physical dominion over women symbolized reason's proper governance over lower intellectual functions and, by extension, intellect's governance over the body, the body's proper subordination to the soul as well as the subordination of the soul's lesser faculties (more integrated with the body) to its highest faculty, reason, could equally serve to legitimize the subordination of women to men. 'Of all the analogies for the soul/body relationship' current in early modern England, Osmond reports that the analogy comparing soul and body to husband and wife is 'the most pervasive and resonant'.[35] Because of the persistent categorization of all women in early modern England according to their marital status – they were either maids, wives, widows, or whores[36] – the husband-wife/soul-body analogy applies to the position of men and women in relation to each other more generally.[37] Significantly, 'the one consistent feature' of the analogy's countless and varied instances is that the body is 'always' 'identified with Eve (woman)', while 'the soul or reason' is 'identified with Adam (man)', since Eve was the one who, 'like sensuality, was attracted to a physical object and thus moved to disobedience'.[38] Two main factors Osmond cites for 'making the woman the body and the man the soul' in English writings, besides the common 'identification of soul and body with Adam and Eve', include the Aristotelian

---

[34]   Lloyd, *Man of Reason*, 30, 32.

[35]   Osmond, *Mutual Accusation*, 157.

[36]   See Mendelson and Crawford, *Women in Early Modern England*, 37, 66.

[37]   As future wives, past wives, or women judged to be 'fallen' because they deviated from the proper progression of maid to wife, in other words, unmarried women were not exempt from this version of gender hierarchy. Even those who chose to remain maids were subject to their fathers, uncles, or brothers, or, if entering a religious vocation, to Christ as divine groom.

[38]   Osmond, *Mutual Accusation*, 157–9.

version of conception that I mentioned earlier[39] and, most important, the fact that this analogy reinforces 'the need for proper subordination' of both wife to husband and body to soul.[40] Even the emerging Puritan model of companionate marriage, which opposed marriage as submission to a tyrannical husband with marriage as a working partnership, argued for a husband's responsibility and respect towards his wife by appealing to Christ's self-sacrificing love for his bride and body, the Church – an analogy that preserves the hierarchy of male over female, divine over earthly.[41]

An entire web of associations and assumptions forms around the conceptual alignment of women with the body and men with the soul. As allegedly more subject to the body than men were, women possessed less reason and lacked control over their passions, determined in large part, of course, by the body's humoural balance. Not only were women more bodily than men, but their bodies were also physiologically inferior to men's bodies, weaker, softer, and more malleable, matching their easily swayed mental constitutions.[42] While most

---

[39]   Mendelson and Crawford, *Women in Early Modern England*, 27, observe that while this version of conception was certainly current, the more 'favoured medical view during the sixteenth and first half of the seventeenth centuries stated that the child was formed from both male and female seed'.

[40]   Osmond, *Mutual Accusation*, 159–60. Osmond provides numerous early modern English examples of the husband-wife/soul-body analogy throughout her study, including, in the section I am quoting from here, passages from Jeremy Taylor ('Sermons Preached at Golden Grove', 1653): 'For the Woman that went before the man in the way of Death, is commanded to follow him in the way of Love ... For then the Soul and Body makes a perfect Man, when the Soul commands wisely, or rules lovingly ... that Body which is its partner and yet the inferior'; and Kenelm Digby ('Sir Kenelm Digby to Sir Edward Stradling', 1663): 'And as the feminine Sex is imperfect, and receiveth perfection from the Masculine; so doth the Body from the Soul, which to it is in lieu of a Male: And as in corporal generations the Female doth afford but gross and passive matter, unto which the male giveth ... prolifical virtue; so in spiritual generations ... the Body administreth only the Organs which, if they were not emplyoyed [sic] by the Soul, would of themselves serve to nothing' (160–61).

[41]   For a full discussion of the Puritan model of companionate marriage and the self-advocating ways in which women writers interpreted and made use of it, see Chapter 1 of Erica Longfellow's *Women and Religious Writing*. See also Maclean, *Renaissance Notion of Woman*, 2.9.2.

[42]   On women's susceptibility to the passions, Michael Schoenfeldt, *Bodies and Selves*, 36, writes that women were 'frequently assumed to be physiologically less capable of the regimens of self-discipline than were men. In *The Secret Miracles of Nature*, Lemnius gives an elaborate humoral explanation for what he believes to be women's innate inability to exercise self-control'. Lemnius claims that women's 'loose, soft and tender' flesh facilitates the fast spread of choler 'all the body over' as soon as it is 'kindled', and that 'the venim and collections of humours that she every month heaps together' are dangerously stirred by anger, which releases noxious vapours that affect the 'Heart and Brain'. Lisa Perfetti (ed.), *Representation of Women's Emotions*, 25, adds that 'thought to be less endowed

early moderns understood their bodies to be very permeable to environmental influences,[43] women's bodies were pathologized as utterly incontinent in comparison to men's, as Gail Kern Paster's important work on humoural theory in *The Body Embarrassed* explores. The 'liquid expressiveness' of the female body, Paster has convincingly demonstrated, discursively connects to the stereotype of women's 'excessive verbal fluency'. 'In both formations', she explains, 'the issue is women's bodily self-control or, more precisely, the representation of a particular kind of uncontrol as a function of gender'.[44] The notion of 'uncontrol' attached to femininity and the body reaches back to Greek philosophical definitions of reason and articulations of the 'form-matter distinction'.[45] These articulations equated 'maleness' with 'a clear, determinate mode of thought' and 'active, determinate form', in contrast to 'femaleness' and 'the unbounded – the vague', 'passive, indeterminate matter'.[46] Ben Jonson's Ursula of *Bartholomew Fair*, whom I discuss in Chapter 1, exemplifies perfectly this notion of female boundlessness and uncontrol. She also exemplifies (albeit eliciting less sympathy than other examples the theatre provides) Gwynne Kennedy's point that women's expressions of emotion could be easily discredited on the grounds that they arose from women's physiological weakness, along with Paster's insight that women's speech could be considered a shameful exposure akin to urinal incontinence and worthy of ridicule.[47] Femininity's associations with passivity and indeterminacy also underlie Francis Bacon's articulation of 'scientific knowledge' as male

---

with the rational faculties that enable one to control the passions, women were considered to be more emotional than men, a belief that persists in many respects today. One might even say that in the medieval way of thinking, emotions *were* female'. Perfetti, 4–5, also explains how humoural theory contributed to the idea that women's bodily constitutions made them more emotional. Maclean, Laqueur, and Paster all cover similar ground in their in-depth studies of how medical theory constructed women's bodies and minds as weaker than men's. Maclean, 'Notion of Woman', 147, notes that 'woman is considered to be inferior to man in that the psychological effects of her cold and moist humours throw doubt on her control of her emotions and her rationality; furthermore, her less robust physique', as defined in medicine, 'predisposes her … to a more protected and less prominent role in the house-hold and in society'. See also Lynette McGrath, *Subjectivity and Women's Poetry*, 40, for a review of how woman's 'dominance by her body inhibits her moral and mental capabilities'. For early modern, non-medical writings that defined the soul as free of passion and aligned passion squarely with the body, see Davies's *Nosce Teipsum*, stanza 25, and Harward's *Discourse Concerning the Soule*, 9–11.

[43]   See Schoenfeldt, *Bodies and Selves*, 8, 14–15, for an explanation of how people in early modern England conceived of their bodies as permeable to environmental influences that needed to be monitored and regulated.

[44]   Gail Kern Paster, *Body Embarrassed*, 25.

[45]   Lloyd, *Man of Reason*, 3.

[46]   Ibid.

[47]   Paster, *Body Embarrassed*, develops this connection in her first chapter on 'Leaky Vessels: The Incontinent Women of City Comedy'. Gwynne Kennedy, *Just Anger*, 8.

'control' over a feminized 'Nature' that might begin as 'mysterious' but is finally 'knowable' and 'manipulable'.[48] The husband-wife analogy finds parallel in many more related analogies for the soul-body relationship current in early modern England that, while adding intriguing nuances, for the most part maintain the division between governor-governed, active-passive, or knower-known that applies to the gendering of soul and body as husband and wife. Osmond's work is particularly useful for gathering together so many examples of these analogies in early modern writings, and even a cursory look at her index gives an idea of the relative consistency of the terms of the divide. Among the entries under body:soul and flesh:spirit analogies are cage:bird; corporal love:spiritual love; grave:body; house:tenant; garden:gardener; lantern:candle; musical instrument:performer; ship:pilot; temple:priest; tool:artificer; and passion:reason, while listed under soul:body are Christ:Church; heaven:earth; King:kingdom; etc.[49]

The following chapters are organized thematically around similar forms of this conventional soul:body dynamic, namely, puppeteer:puppet, tamer:tamed, ghost:haunted, and observer:spectacle. These analogies are both at work in and challenged by the representations of women in the plays and masques I investigate. While these pairings are not among those explicit soul-body analogies Osmond has collected from early modern writings, thematically they certainly align with her findings as well as with the prevalent early modern concepts of the soul-body dynamic discussed above. The puppeteer-puppet relationship illustrates both the early modern version of Platonic dualism, which viewed the body as passive material animated by the superior soul, and the Aristotelian idea of the body as a tool or instrument through which the soul-as-artist can express itself and interact with the world. In his comprehensive study of puppetry in the period and beyond, Scott Cutler Shershow also identifies the puppet as representing the spirit-flesh opposition and, moreover, as 'resembl[ing] the cultural image of Woman as ... associated with the body in its binary opposition to the spirit', a connection that Chapter 1 explores at length.[50] The relationship between a 'tamer' and the person being 'tamed' or brought under control reflects the influential Platonic notion of the soul as the rightful governor of a body that can often be unruly (linked, for instance, to the wild horse representing appetite in the chariot analogy). The ghost:haunted relationship allows for interaction between a disembodied spirit and someone who remains in the flesh in a way that visually and thematically hearkens back to the soul-body dialogues of the early sixteenth century, a genre that, as Osmond's extensive work on it discusses, influenced seventeenth-century dramatic themes before being explicitly revisited later in the seventeenth century by poets such as Andrew Marvell.[51] Finally, the interplay between observer and spectacle resonates with that of soul and body in that discernment and judgement were located in

---

[48]   Lloyd, *Man of Reason*, 10–17.
[49]   Osmond, *Mutual Accusation*, 273–4.
[50]   Scott Cutler Shershow, *Puppets and 'Popular' Culture*, 72.
[51]   Osmond, *Mutual Accusation*.

the rational or higher part of the soul, while the material pleasures of spectacle appealed to the 'lower' passions and lusts of the body and also included the body as itself an attractive spectacle. The soul-body dynamic underpins each of these very theatrical and, as each chapter explores, heavily gendered relationships.

In highlighting these four distinct yet related theatrical relationships my intention is not to argue by analogy, a practice that can indeed be tricky and slippery, but to reflect the reality that the soul-body dynamic itself was primarily understood and expressed through analogy. The richly figurative language of the booming commercial theatre, the popular emblem book tradition, the inventive poetic use of metaphor later distinguished as metaphysical conceit – all part of the innovative literary culture that characterized the period – suggest that people in early modern England were generally quite accustomed to thinking through analogy. The soul-body dynamic operated on gender ideology mainly through the widely familiar soul-body/husband-wife comparison (outlined above and explored in greater depth through the following chapters), and each of these four pairings functions, in the plays or masques under consideration, as a variation on, or nuanced expression of, this central marriage analogy.

The Feminized Soul: An Exception to the Rule?

I want to address a question that, by this point, will have come up for someone familiar with explicit references to the soul in early English literature, and especially in devotional poetry: don't most writers, poets, and even clergy always use feminine pronouns to refer to the soul, and don't they usually depict the soul as a female figure? And do these references not overturn the claim that the body is most often feminized in contrast to a soul that is masculinized? Depictions of and references to the soul as female are certainly conventional, but often occur when the writer is considering the soul either in isolation or in relationship to Christ. The soul as female, in other words, tends not to find an explicit contrast in emphatically masculine physicality or bodiliness.[52] The literary convention of making the soul feminine rarely produces empowering representations of women as possessing superior intellect, morality, or other faculties of the soul, in the way that the association of women with the body connects to such disadvantageous

---

[52] A notable exception may be George Herbert's 'Church-Monuments', ll. 1, 7, in which the speaker describes his soul as repairing 'to *her* devotion' while his body learns to 'spell *his* elements' and 'find *his* birth', but the pronoun 'his' might also simply be intended as a neutral pronoun, as 'his' was frequently used in the way we would now use 'its' (emphases added). The reference to the body as 'it' instead of 'he' in the preceding line supports the likelihood that 'his' is a neutral possessive pronoun here. Just as the soul is gendered feminine when considered in isolation, Osmond, *Mutual Accusation*, 167, points out that the rare identifications of women with the soul in Jacobean drama are 'normally limited to situations where they are viewed alone, apart from the context of their relationship with men'.

representations of women as weak, irrational, and lacking self-control. The biblical notion of God as 'father, bridegroom, king', and of 'the human soul and the church' as 'daughter, bride, and consort',[53] leads John Donne, 'in his sacred poetry and prose', to consider masculinity a kind of 'spiritual liability', as Elizabeth Hodgson explains,[54] but not so much because women themselves were somehow inherently more in tune with the soul than were men based on their biological makeup. Rather, while Donne sees the 'conventional values of feminine submission and interdependence' as necessary in an individual's relationship with God, he maintains a 'distinction between "women" and "the feminine"' in his self-representations.[55] For Donne the soul's femininity, then, has less to do with an exalting of women's spiritual affinity or capacity than with an affirmation of the feminine as a marker of subordination, weakness, inferiority – qualities that are desirable and appropriate for everyone in relationship to God, but only for women on a practical, everyday basis. Beyond Donne, as a literary convention the feminization of the soul remains subject to male control. In her comprehensive survey of imaginative depictions of the soul in Western culture, Osmond notes that despite the varied characteristics and 'multiple roles' of the feminine soul – she may be 'a rather remote figure, awe-inspiring in her beauty and purity', or 'of the more earthly feminine, seductive and approachable, but still refined beyond the merely sexual', and she might appear to 'inspire, advise, reproach', or 'condemn' – one thing remains the same. Clarifying that she is 'not using the word "men" in the inclusive sense', Osmond asserts that 'the feminine soul comes to *men*. They painted the pictures and wrote the texts'.[56] This tradition suggests that the feminization of the soul is wrapped up in male attempts to define or manage the very concept of the soul, to render visible and facilitate comprehension of – and thus to gain some control over – a complex and mysterious entity.[57]

In addition to being connected to male artistic control, the feminization of the soul might, paradoxically, stem from the association of women with the body. The soul is not the only abstract concept to be represented through female personification. The traditional representation of several emotions and virtues also personifies them as female figures, and James Paxson suggests that the gendering

---

[53]   Theresa M. DiPasquale, *Refiguring the Sacred Feminine*, 1. In n. 2 of this page, DiPasquale offers a useful reference to multiple old and new testament passages in which the figuring of the soul as daughter and bride appear.

[54]   Elizabeth M.A. Hodgson, *Gender and the Sacred Self in John Donne*, 13.

[55]   Ibid., 14–15.

[56]   Rosalie Osmond, *Imagining the Soul*, 47.

[57]   Also connected to the feminization of the soul as a measure of artistic control is the suggestion in Paul Martin, 'The Body in the Realm of Desire', 102–3, that this gendering was invoked to avoid homoerotic tones for men expressing desire for Christ. Jonathan Goldberg (ed.), *Queering the Renaissance*, however, cautions against critically reading homoeroticism in devotional expressions as something that writers sought to avoid.

of the body as female lies at the root of such feminizations of abstract concepts. As Lisa Perfetti lucidly summarizes this point in her introduction to Paxson's essay:

> the tendency to personify abstract concepts like emotions as female came from the deep structure of classical rhetoric that hinges on a series of associations: since the body is female, and since the use of rhetorical figures is associated with the body because they give form to (or 'embody') abstract thought, then rhetorical figures are associated with femininity.[58]

For these reasons – the feminization of abstract concepts and ideals as circling back to notions of embodiment as female; the feminization of the soul as a measure of artistic control; and the distinction between feminine subjection as an ideal attitude to assume towards God versus feminine subjection as a consequence of real women's supposed inferiority to men – literary references to the soul as female fail to significantly contradict the strong cultural alignment of women with the body and of men with the soul and the patriarchal subordination of women that this alignment underpinned.[59]

Destabilizing the Hierarchy

Articulations of the overall relationship between soul and body, spirit and matter that ran counter to the conventional structuring of the relationship as a hierarchical division, however, were also available. Continuing religious belief in the eventual resurrection of the body at the Last Judgement asserted the body's value, along with the soul, as an integral part of the eternal self.[60] Writings on childbirth and nursing record the belief that 'maternal imagination' during pregnancy could affect the child's physical appearance, and that a child imbibed some of its mother's (or wet nurse's) moral disposition along with her breast milk.[61] The fluidity between material and immaterial apparent in these notions of motherly influence contravenes the notion that women only passively supply matter to their children,

---

[58] Perfetti, *Representation of Women's Emotions*, 4.

[59] This general claim is not to deny that the representation of the soul and of other abstract concepts as feminine could sometimes create an opening for the characterization of femininity as powerful and not subject to male control. The closest example I have found occurs in Jane Anger, *Jane Anger Her Protection for Women*, B2v, 'if we women be so perillous cattell as they terme us, I marvell that the Gods made not Fidelitie as well a man, as they created her a woman, and all the morall vertues of their masculine sex, as of the feminine kinde, except their Deities knewe that there was some soveraity in us women, which could not be in them men'.

[60] Caroline Walker Bynum's *Resurrection of the Body in Western Christianity* provides a fascinating and comprehensive account of the history of belief in the physical body's resurrection after death, investigating its many nuanced articulations, developments, impetuses, and implications.

[61] Mendelson and Crawford, *Women in Early Modern England*, 28–9.

while men pass on the soul. And yet the blurring of a division between material and immaterial in this case can become a means to tack blame onto the mother for a child's poor disposition or, perhaps, abnormal appearance;[62] it does not serve to dislodge the association between women and inferiority.

Nonetheless, while I have used the terms 'divide', 'dichotomy', or 'hierarchy' to describe the dominant version of the soul-body relationship as a masculinized soul meant to govern a feminized body, in the title of this study and in the discussions that follow, I favour the term 'soul-body dynamic' in order to encompass this pervasive model as well as alternative versions that pushed against it and that also circulated in early modern culture. Artistic play with the soul-body dynamic in early modern poetry, prose, and my current focus, drama, reveals a wide range of attitudes towards soul and body. Some of these attitudes rehearse traditional gender hierarchies while others, I argue, often within the same play or masque, open up space for more flexible, less misogynistic understandings of gendered relationships, regardless of authorial intention. The possibility that literary engagement with the soul-body dynamic can engender more positive views of women has received attention in women's writing from Lynette McGrath, who has discovered a tendency for women to invest the body with subjectivity in a way that responds to the increasing association of women with the body by emphasizing the body's own complex wisdom as opposed to its inferiority.[63] The connection between dramatic treatments of the soul-body dynamic and representations of women, however, has not yet served as a focal point for early modern literary criticism.

While in early modern thought the soul generally took precedence over the body, the reverse is true in current early modern scholarship. In choosing the soul-body dynamic as my focal point in a study on dramatic representations of women, I am indebted to McGrath's findings and to scholars such as Paster, Lloyd, Laqueur, Maclean, Mendelson, Crawford, and others who have drawn attention to the ways women were so persistently associated with the body or relegated to bodily roles in society and to the ways that body was understood and pathologized. Their work is part of what Ewan Fernie and Ramona Wray identify, in their assessment of the recent critical landscape in Renaissance studies, as 'a wider movement in the humanities, from the spiritual to the material', a 'shift' signalled by the body's place at 'centre stage' in criticism.[64] While this shift has been immensely productive, the recent scholarly emphasis on the body and materiality tends to downplay early modern concepts of the soul, even when the relationship between the material and immaterial is broached. When Michael Schoenfeldt considers the relationship between 'physiology and inwardness' in his study of early modern *Bodies and Selves*, for instance, he focuses on corporeality and favours terms like 'inwardness', 'mind', 'emotions', or 'psychological interiority', without always

---

62   Ibid.
63   See, for instance, McGrath, *Subjectivity and Women's Poetry*, 47, 64.
64   Ewan Fernie, Ramona Wray, et al. (eds), *Reconceiving the Renaissance*, 9.

making clear where early modern concepts of the soul fit into this terminology.[65] In her study of early modern inwardness, Katharine Eisaman Maus points out that for 'many new-historicist and cultural materialist critics', 'soul' (along with the aligned terms 'privacy', 'inwardness', and 'subjectivity') is a suspicious term that 'beg[s] to be debunked'.[66] The translation of the soul into terms we are critically more comfortable with, however, is problematic, given that, as Lisa Hopkins rightly observes, 'the intensity of the early seventeenth-century interest in the body by no means precluded an equally eager interest in the soul'.[67] Even more problematically, the critical elision of the soul in discussions of inwardness and subjectivity risks losing sight of how persistently early modern culture gendered the very components a predominantly Christian society would conceive of as constituting the self. One of the useful insights that Maus's work offers, for instance, is that a 'connection between a challenge to authority and a highly developed sense of personal inwardness is … intrinsic',[68] but, as McGrath's readings of women's writings suggest, inwardness might not be part of female subjectivity in remotely the same way it might be part of male subjectivity. My study is more concerned with representations of women than with theories of early modern subjectivity, to which both Maus and Schoenfeldt contribute. Representation, however, can both reflect and suggest new subject-positions for women.

While the present critical landscape requires that we avoid the pitfall of reproducing the early modern moral convention of prioritizing the soul, my study addresses an emerging need to resist skewing our perspective of the period by giving precedence to corporeality to an extent that does not accurately reflect the balance of early modern concerns. Stepping back from the body to reassess the full complexity of seventeenth-century assumptions about the soul and body together is especially important for adding to our knowledge of the cultural limitations and possibilities that women faced. The following chapters work to redefine one of the period's most pervasive analogies for conceptualizing women and their relations to men as more complex and shifting than criticism has previously assumed. Through sustained focus on the soul-body dynamic I seek to open a new interpretive framework for reading representations of women, adding to the ongoing feminist reevaluation of the kinds of power women might actually wield despite the patriarchal strictures of their culture. Finally, by analyzing dramatic texts from the late sixteenth and early seventeenth centuries, each chapter demonstrates the importance of drama to scholarly considerations of the soul-body dynamic, which habitually turn to devotional works, sermons, and philosophical and religious treatises to elucidate this relationship.

---

[65]   Schoenfeldt does refer explicitly to early modern treatments of the opposition between 'body and soul' or 'spirit and matter', but in isolated sections of his study (6–11, 40–41, 56–7, 60, 77–9, 98–102) as part of, but not central to, a consideration of 'physiology and inwardness'.

[66]   Katharine Eisaman Maus, *Inwardness and Theatre*, 27.

[67]   Lisa Hopkins, *Female Hero*, 118.

[68]   Maus, *Inwardness and Theatre*, 70. On the connection between interiority and resistance to authority, see also Elizabeth Hanson, *Discovering the Subject*, 17.

Why Male-Authored, Secular Drama?

My focus on Jacobean drama aims, in part, to highlight that the gendered soul-body dynamic plays a role in representations of and attitudes towards women beyond literature that engages explicitly and centrally with this relationship (such as devotional poetry, for instance, or philosophical and religious treatises). Theatre necessarily engages the interplay between material and immaterial more broadly, often drawing attention to the fluidity and tensions between the two. This quality of theatre makes it particularly fitting for an investigation into the cultural values inflecting the soul-body dynamic and their impact on representations of women. Theatre constantly conveys the immaterial, whether emotions, dreams, or departed spirits, for instance, in very material ways, and conversely conjures certain material events through onstage storytelling or chorus narration as though to enhance their impact by leaving them to the audience's imagination. My first chapter elaborates on this interplay by discussing the elusive, ghost-like qualities of Gloriana's very material skull in *The Revenger's Tragedy*.

In concentrating on dramatic representations of women, I share Alison Findlay's position that:

> the absence of women from [theatre] companies does not mean that professional Renaissance drama is an all-male activity. The meanings of plays presented on the commercial stages were not produced solely by the writers and actors. Spectators were an integral element in Renaissance drama … [and] we do know that women made up a significant part of Renaissance theatre audiences.[69]

Women were not entirely excluded from participation in these representations and, indeed, their own writings bear the imprint of the same patriarchal ideology that the stage reflects. My focus on Jacobean drama for the angle it offers into my topic, then, does not mean to privilege these representations over women's self-presentations, but rather to produce new readings of the plays that might be productively put into conversation with female-authored texts. I am intrigued, for instance, by Jacqueline Broad's argument that particularly women writers and philosophers of the second half of the seventeenth century and into the early eighteenth century reject post-Cartesian dualism in favour of a concept of flesh and spirit as more complexly integrated.[70] Dualism, obviously, does not make its

---

[69]   Alison Findlay, *A Feminist Perspective on Renaissance Drama*, 1. Naomi Conn Liebler (ed.), *Female Tragic Hero*, 3, also develops the point that 'the success of any play required the receptiveness of women', drawing on previous scholarship by Findlay, Stephen Orgel, Jean Howard, and Linda Woodbridge, and refuting the argument that 'male authorship definitively precludes female heroism or that men can only write the feminine inimically', as well as the ideas that 'experience can only be known and represented from within a specific sexual identity, that there are irreconcilable differences between male and female "ways of knowing", that the female characters written by Shakespeare and his contemporaries are only a male fantasy of the female and can only be represented as "Other"'.

[70]   Jacqueline Broad, *Women Philosophers*, 10–12.

first entrance with Descartes, and I would posit that the seeds of what women such as Margaret Cavendish more explicitly and fully articulated later in the century are already present in earlier dramatic play with soul-body concepts and representations of women, although my current study can only take a step in the direction of making such a claim conclusively.

In addition to these compelling reasons for turning to drama to elucidate the connection between the soul-body dynamic and gender representation, namely, drama's own composite nature, comprised of material and immaterial elements, and the need to consider and appeal to the women who made up a significant portion of the audiences, another reason presents itself in the fact that attacks on theatre in post-Reformation England were often concerned with some aspect of theatre's materiality. Just as views of women's moral and intellectual inferiority to men hinged upon women's supposedly stronger ties to the body, views of theatre as a corrupting influence hinged upon theatre's bodiliness, or its appeal to the body. Indeed, Puritan anti-theatricalists frequently describe the theatre as itself feminine and as rendering its participants and spectators effeminate. Discussing William Prynne's 1633 *Histriomastix* as a culmination of the growing anti-theatrical attack that accompanied the institutionalization of professional theatre (with the building of playhouses, the crown's protection, and government regulations) and as an example of 'the tendencies of most antitheatrical polemic from 1575 to the closing of the theaters', Jonas Barish observes:

> emphasis falls heavily on two sorts of offences: on sports and games and festive activities – on anything that gives pleasure and is patently designed as recreation – and even more obsessively on sexuality and effeminacy, as though to underscore the author's fearful aversion to anything – dancing, love-making, hair-curling, elegant attire – that might suggest active or interested sexuality, this being equated with femininity, with weakness, with the yielding to feeling, and consequently with the destruction of all assured props and boundaries.[71]

Theatre – with its portrayal of intense emotions, its elaborate costumes, makeup, poetic language, music, dancing, and gesture – gave pleasure to the senses. Borrowing from Plato's objections to theatre (and to poetry more generally), which depended upon his understanding of the soul-body relationship, early modern anti-theatricalists faulted theatre for a disordering impact on spectators: it stirred and indulged passion and desire, belonging to the lower faculties of the soul and linked to the body, thus distracting from the higher part of the soul and disturbing the soul's rightful government of the body, reason's proper control of the passions.[72]

---

[71] Jonas Barish, *Antitheatrical Prejudice*, 83, 85. For more on anti-theatrical attacks on theatre as effeminate and effeminizing, see also Chapter 3, n. 18.

[72] Within a comprehensive explanation of the 'Platonic foundation' for early modern anti-theatrical prejudice, Barish, *Antitheatrical Prejudice*, 9–11, discusses this connection between Plato's notion of the soul's hierarchy and his stance against poetry in general.

Puritan anti-theatricalism, of course, formed part of a broader religious iconoclasm directed against Catholic devotional uses of imagery and ritual. In a consideration of two influential Reformist texts published in 1563 – the homily on idolatry designed for 'delivery in churches throughout the country' and 'officially sanctioned' by the monarchy, and the second edition of John Foxe's *Acts and Monuments* – Susan Zimmerman explains that, 'considered jointly, these propagandistic texts articulated a new and strongly felt Protestant anxiety about the body – put simply, a need to envisage its materiality, like that of the idol, as dead',[73] or, in other words, as something to which we should not accord value. And, 'in an important sense', Zimmerman argues, early modern English 'theatre developed *as theatre* in continual tension with a pervasive Protestant ideology that sought to revise the conceptual framework for apprehending the material body'. Zimmerman finds, for instance, that 'the new theatrical industry' did not 'shrink from examining the issue of idolatry in its own right by means of corporeal representations'.[74] Early modern dramatists demonstrate a self-consciousness and often a sense of ambivalence or conflict about the materiality of their craft. Although not addressing explicitly the issue of materiality, critics such as Barish and Ellen Mackay explore, in different ways, theatre's self-consciousness in response to its detractors. Barish offers readings of Shakespeare both championing and villainizing theatricality in the sense of multiple self-transformations, and of Jonson's even deeper ambivalence about the 'theatrical', which involved, among other things, contempt for audiences he viewed as frequenting the theatre only to 'make spectacles of themselves' and 'compete with the play'.[75] Mackay, drawing from Stephen Gosson's *Schoole of Abuse* and Thomas Heywood's *Apology for Actors*, finds a 'surprising consensus' that 'for the theater's defenders no less than for its antagonists … the performances that pass through the playhouse impact their beholders like gunfire'. For Mackay, acknowledging the theatre's ability to cause 'hurt' also acknowledges that 'what happens on stage counts; if sometimes for the worse, then surely also for the better'.[76]

Despite our awareness of this theatrical self-consciousness that developed alongside vehement hostility towards the theatre, and despite our knowledge about similarities between attacks on the theatre for its materiality on one hand, and negative views of women for their bodiliness on the other, we have not yet explored the connection that might exist – regardless of authorial intention – between onstage vindications of theatricality and more positive stage portrayals of women. We might expect that rather than condemning the physicality of their craft along with their critics, dramatists would be more inclined to invest in refiguring the soul-body dynamic in the ways I am arguing for in this book – in ways, that is, that carried repercussions for representations of gender as

---

[73]   Susan Zimmerman, *Early Modern Corpse*, 46.
[74]   Ibid., 90.
[75]   Barish, *Antitheatrical Prejudice*, 127–33.
[76]   Ellen Mackay, *Persecution, Plague, and Fire*, 8–10, 19–20.

well as for representations of theatricality itself. In the plays and masques this book analyzes, the more positive depictions of women – or the departures from strains of misogyny also present in the play – repeatedly coincide with a male character coming to a transformative realization through explicitly theatrical means. *Bartholomew Fair*'s Busy is cured of his hypocrisy by a puppet show when all else fails; Petruccio in *The Tamer Tamed* reforms his notion of his role as husband only after his wife stages a series of public performances that expose his shortcomings to the community; *The Lady's Tragedy*'s Tyrant, although an abuser of theatricality's power, is finally conquered by a theatrical display that restores order to the kingdom. Vindice, too, employs theatrical display to conquer a corrupt political ruler in *The Revenger's Tragedy*, but he also undervalues the material and misses a theatrical cue to his own demise. Queen Anna's masques do not feature a male character coming to a transformative realization in the same way, but they do constitute in themselves a strategic use of theatricality to effect a particular realization in James or in the audience about Anna and her ladies. These instances, which the following chapters explore more fully, suggest a justification of theatre's materiality in post-Reformation culture based on its didactic efficacy. And in each case, a reevaluation of materiality and theatricality corresponds with a reconsideration of misogynistic stereotypes about women.

The plays and masques this book concentrates on are from the Jacobean period, a period in which dramatic focus on female characters increased significantly.[77] My first chapter on puppetry in Middleton's *The Revenger's Tragedy* and Jonson's *Bartholomew Fair* draws a connection between the gender-coded soul-body dynamic and the gendering of the relationship between puppeteer and puppet. I argue that the central performance of puppetry in these two plays noted for their

---

[77] Liebler, *Female Tragic Hero*, 20–23, points out the increase in plays focusing on tragic female heroes during the Jacobean period: 'From Elizabeth's succession to her death, a period of enormous dramatic production, fewer than 30 tragedies appear whose titles are women's names … ; most of these 30 are listed as "closet" plays, not intended for performance, and about half of them … are lost. For about 20 of those first 30 years, nearly all of these female-titled tragedies represent women from Greco-Roman tragedy. … Then, during the last decade of Elizabeth's reign, we begin to get original drama featuring female protagonists. … Not until the Jacobeans, with some 18 instances between 1604 and 1625, does the female tragic protagonist command the stage and the page as the titular hero'. Lisa Hopkins, *Female Hero*, 2, also claims that 'The rise of the strong female hero, who may be in some respects a victim but is also an initiator, emerges as a widespread phenomenon in the period from about 1610, when we find a rush of female tragic protagonists on the English stage'. Hopkins suggests that 'the rise of the female protagonist' links to 'particular and highly contested debates within early modern culture and drama in England, including changing ideas about the relationship between bodies and souls and between men's bodies and women's, marriage and mothering, the law, religion and the nature of theatrical representation itself'. I will be considering comedies and masques alongside tragedies, but Hopkins's and Liebler's observations about an increased interest in female figures in tragedy, I think, suggest a definite cultural shift that is relevant to Jacobean drama more broadly.

rampant misogyny calls into question the misogynistic treatment of women. Much as Donne demonstrates his wit in Problem VII at the expense of women in general, *The Revenger's Tragedy*'s Vindice uses his dead fiançée's skull as a visual prop for his witty speeches, assuming control over the feminine and the material to showcase his own intelligence. *Bartholomew Fair* culminates in a hilarious puppet show that thematically reflects men's treatment of women as property throughout the play. Although in *theory* puppetry – an active wit imposing meaning upon and animating passive material – works as an analogy for the dominant version of the soul-body dynamic, I contend that in *performance* puppetry productively troubles this version. The appearance of actual puppets onstage tends to captivate and fascinate the audience in a way that parodies and unsettles a hierarchical distinction between spirit and flesh, controller and controlled. Through puppets that escape the puppeteer's control, material that overpowers its animating spirit or wit, each play stages the consequences – fatal in one case and humiliating in the other – of attempting to control women and of refusing to learn from the material. I discuss the feminized puppet's uncanny energy as something that emerges from, and yet troubles, patriarchal assumptions about women. The chapter embeds readings of both plays' puppetry within an historical account of English puppetry in religious and popular entertainments that highlights the puppet's associations with femininity and with rebellion. I suggest the broader relevance of the chapter's readings by making comparative reference to the impulse to puppet women, both literally and metaphorically, in a variety of other contemporary plays, including Shakespeare's *The Taming of the Shrew*.

While the first chapter considers how the signifying force of onstage material can wordlessly reshape the soul-body dynamic (and its impact on thinking about gender), Chapter 2 examines a more immaterial form of engagement with the dynamic. I argue that Fletcher's *The Tamer Tamed* demonstrates a critical awareness of the gendered division of soul and body as a rhetorical construct employed to subordinate women and to justify male authority. Beyond exposing the gendering of soul and body as a rhetorical weapon wielded against women, Fletcher's play suggests that women can meet this rhetorical construct with new rhetoric more advantageous to their sex. I read Maria's flexible new rhetoric in response to her husband's attempts to puppet her (as he puppeted Katharina during his past life in Shakespeare's *The Taming of the Shrew*) as doubly radical in terms of unsettling gender assumptions. First, Maria's rhetoric draws upon contemporary theory about the soul to insist on a connection between her will and her soul. This insistence recasts female wilfulness – stereotypically a sign of wild irrationality and a need to be tamed – as a sign of female intelligence and rational desire. Second, Fletcher's Maria taps into the early modern discourse of rhetoric, and specifically the anxieties surrounding rhetoric's reliance on an understanding of emotion, suggesting that women possess a natural capacity to be the best rhetors, despite their exclusion from formal rhetorical training. The implications are far-reaching in light of the rhetor's aim of gaining power through influencing the wills (and souls) of others. I explore the gender implications of Maria's shifting rhetoric, which sometimes blurs and at other times rigidly demarcates body and soul.

Expanding on ideas about the feminine uncanny that I develop in Chapter 1, as well as on ideas about women's relationship to rhetoric in Chapter 2, Chapter 3 examines a female tragic hero whose strong rhetoric is violently separated from her body when she becomes a ghost. Middleton's *The Lady's Tragedy* takes to the extreme the connection (discussed in Chapter 2) that Fletcher's Maria makes between her will and her soul, staging a strong-willed and witty woman who literally becomes nothing but soul. The Lady takes charge of her fate, competently directs those around her, and acts as the source of reason, but the play disembodies her assertive voice. I argue that this transformation only slightly mitigates the threat the Lady poses to the patriarchal ideal of male authority over women. The play does suggest that a woman's attempts to govern people and direct events independently from male authority end up violently detaching her from her body, sacrificing the private relationships dependent upon that body. In one sense, the resulting ghostly attempts to direct people's actions are ineffective in their entire dependence on the willingness of others to listen and obey. In another sense, though, this weakness is more of a strength and offers an incisive critique of the origins and responsibilities of governmental power and authority. I demonstrate how cultural concepts of the soul-body dynamic add depth to this critique, especially concerning the implications of juxtaposing disembodied female authority with a male tyrant consumed by bodily lust. I argue that *The Lady's Tragedy* reverses the usual gendering of soul and body, exposing the male prerogative to govern as a violent but well-disguised usurpation of women's rightful authority over themselves.

Each of the chapters considers, to a degree, moments onstage that collapse the idea of a hierarchical divide between soul and body. The primary focus on the material in Chapter 1 and the concentration on rhetoric and the immaterial in Chapters 2 and 3, however, become most fully integrated in the final chapter. Chapter 4 examines masques in which Queen Anna performed with her ladies, giving particular attention to Daniel's *The Vision of the Twelve Goddesses* and *Tethys Festival*, with supporting discussion of Jonson's *The Masque of Blackness* and *The Masque of Queens*. I argue that in these masques, the performing female body comes to visually and thematically represent the soul. This bodily representation of the soul challenges women's exclusion from political government. It thus constitutes a political statement that does not hinge on sexual transgressiveness, a topic that past feminist masque criticism has foregrounded. My interpretation further departs from previous feminist criticism on masque by reading Jonson's and Daniel's theorizations of masque structure, which they explicitly compare to the soul-body dynamic, as complementing rather than contradicting the women's physical performance. I draw on three main contexts to support my argument: I discuss the soul-body dynamic as a foundational support for the analogous king-subject and husband-wife relationships, a support that King

James himself mobilizes in *Basilikon Doron*; I bring attention to the persistent connection between movement and the soul in various early modern treatises on the soul, developing the significance of this connection to themes of agency in the masques' narratives; and I consider early modern theories of dance as a form of language and rhetoric. In addition to picking up the book's threads on rhetoric and on governmental authority, this chapter pushes further my consideration of Renaissance thematic and performative links between women and puppetry. I argue that the motif of divine possession that Daniel employs in his masques renews the puppetry motif to produce a more positive depiction of women.

By focusing on two tragedies, two comedies, and a small selection of masques, I endeavour to provide thorough and nuanced readings of each work's representation of women in light of body-soul concepts and, at the same time, to demonstrate that this connection between body-soul concepts and representations of women spans a variety of theatrical genres. With the exception of Fletcher's play, each work I examine, moreover, has been read as forwarding particularly negative views of women. Courtly dance, especially in masque, enacted and reinforced existing social codes stipulating women's subordination and deference to men and stressing women's position as objects for the active male gaze.[78] In *The Revenger's Tragedy* two female characters' dead bodies suffer exposure as sensational spectacles subject to the male gaze and to male interpretation, and despite the virtue that Vindice's sister demonstrates – echoing Gloriana's actions in life – the witty protagonist delivers a litany of cleverly turned misogynistic claims in connection with Gloriana, his mother, and women in general that do not meet with the slightest verbal challenge or contestation. *Bartholomew Fair* presents, in Ursula the pig-woman, the most extreme literary example of the association between women and flesh that I can think of. And even while Fletcher's Maria is appealingly proto-feminist, Petruccio unleashes a full arsenal of misogynistic jokes and threats to the amusement of his peers and the audience.[79] In each of these works, an underlying rethinking of the body-soul dynamic, I argue, functions as a strong undercurrent of criticism to effectively challenge such expressions of misogyny and trouble the patriarchal ideal of female subordination, as well as to open up alternative, often more positive readings of the women represented.

---

[78]   See, for instance, M. Bella Mirabella, 'Mute Rhetorics', 415, 424–5, and Clare McManus, *Women on the Renaissance Stage*, 55.

[79]   In a performance of *Tamer* at the Theatre Erindale (2009), the male characters often onstage with Petruccio would always laugh and jeer appreciatively at the insults Petruccio hurled at Maria, whose counter-remarks were boosted by laughter from her female allies. The audience laughed at the insults from both sides, perhaps encouraged by the onstage laughter.

Chapter 1
Puppeteer and Puppet

Gender and Early Modern Puppetry

> Belike you mean to make a puppet of me.
> – Katharina in *The Taming of the Shrew* (4.3.103)

Puppetry brings to a sharp focus the interrelationship between representations of women and cultural inscriptions of the soul-body dynamic. This chapter locates Vindice's dark puppetry of Gloriana's skull in Middleton's *The Revenger's Tragedy* (1606–1607) and the comic puppetry in Jonson's *Bartholomew Fair* (1614) within the contexts of the puppet's cultural history in early modern England and the puppet's facility as a metaphor for the soul-body relationship. I argue for a crucial and productive difference between how the puppet signifies as metaphor and how it signifies as performative object. Metaphorically speaking, to call someone a puppet in seventeenth-century England amounted to an insult, as it would today, insinuating mental vacuousness, superficiality, and an inability to act unless under someone else's control. One significant difference in early modern usage is that the term 'puppet' was much more gendered than in today's usage. This metaphorical reading of the puppet as a sign for the empty, the subordinate, the controlled does not, however, translate to the puppet onstage. The performing puppet often holds a special fascination for audiences and an uncanny capacity to signal meaning apart from the puppeteer's intentions. In light of the feminization of the puppet as it overlaps with the feminization of the body in the soul-body relationship, this difference between the metaphorical invocation of the puppet and actual puppet performance – or, to put it differently, the onstage puppet's disruptive signifying power – holds positive implications for the representation of women more broadly. In both *The Revenger's Tragedy* and *Bartholomew Fair* puppetry presents a misogynistic view of women and yet, in some ways, works to overturn this view.

The appearance of puppets on the commercial playhouse stage is not the same thing as a puppet performance on a street corner or at a fair. Scott Cutler Shershow describes the human theatre's relationship with puppet theatre as one of 'cultural subordination' and 'appropriation', observing uses of the puppet 'as metaphor, metadramatic device, or discursive standard of reference – by writers who also define puppet theater as a mode of culture somehow "lower", less literary and more popular, than their own texts'.[1] This perception of puppet theatre as 'a debased version of the human stage' comes in part from its location

---

[1]   Scott Cutler Shershow, *Puppets*, 44, see 44–8.

'in the marginal social spheres of carnival, fairground, and marketplace', but it also comes from a 'master system of representation … conceived as a descent of primary to secondary, "truth" to image'. In other words, 'the puppet would be to the player as the player is to the author: one step closer to formless materiality, and one step farther from that postulated if irretrievable "truth" from which is said to spring the multitudinous re-creations of theatrical performance'.[2] Shershow's explanation returns us to the Platonic hierarchy of true form over imperfect copy, spirit over matter, with the puppet, of course, as copy and matter. Perhaps the main difference between puppets in motions[3] performed at markets or in the streets and puppets on the playhouse stage has to do with the enactment of this hierarchy on the playhouse stage.

On the playhouse stage puppets were not the clear main attraction, but were subordinated as a thematic complement to broader issues in the unfolding human drama. Puppets in motions at festivals and fairs, moreover, communicated to their audiences in large, broad strokes; they wore exaggerated facial features and spoke rather simple, roughshod verse, as discussed further on. The playhouse appropriation of puppet performance, however, sets puppetry in critical or interrogative relation with other elements of the play's wider narrative in a way that allows the puppet to convey meaning more subtly than it likely would in a motion – even if the puppet looked and behaved much as it would in a fairground performance. A play's juxtaposition of the act of puppetry with the various other relationships and actions it depicts, I posit, adds to this subtlety by fully exploiting the puppet's metaphorical significance alongside its effect as a performative object – a metaphorical significance that draws on the puppet's 'low' or debased status. In this chapter, I accept George Speaight's definition of a puppet as 'an inanimate figure moved by human agency',[4] a definition that excludes automata, but is flexible enough to allow for a consideration of unconventional puppets that appear on the playhouse stage – such as a human skull in *The Revenger's Tragedy* – within the context of the cultural associations surrounding puppetry as a familiar form of street entertainment.

To set up my discussion of what might be at stake for women in theatre's invocation of puppetry, I turn first to Katharina's recognition in *The Taming of the Shrew* (1592–1594) that her new husband is like a puppet master. At a point when she is exasperated at being denied a desirable gown and cap through Petruchio's pretences that the tailor has marred them, Katharina's voiced suspicion that Petruchio must want to make her his puppet is a shrewd one. Beyond referring to how Petruchio is asserting control over her appearance by refusing her the choice of her own garments, Katharina's puppet metaphor points to something even more sinister in Petruchio's behaviour. Petruchio might initially imagine his

---

    [2]   Ibid, 48.

    [3]   A term referring to both puppets and puppet plays. See George Speaight, *English Puppet Theatre*, 54–5.

    [4]   Ibid., 22.

'peremptory' nature meeting the 'proud-minded' Katharina as 'two raging fires' that 'consume the thing that feeds their fury' when they meet, or as 'extreme gusts' of wind that 'blow out fire and all',[5] but clearly he is not interested in a mutual subduing. All the consuming or blowing out must take place within Katharina. Petruchio expects his will to replace Katharina's as the animating spark of her behaviour, and even take precedence over her own perceptions. This expectation is evident in his dizzying progression from deciding his wife's apparel to insisting that before he and Katharina will journey to her sister's wedding, 'It shall be what o'clock I say it is' and not what time Katharina knows it is (4.3.191). In Plato's division of the soul, which remained influential into the seventeenth century, the will or 'spirited element' is one of the soul's faculties, the 'natural ally' of reason in the *Phaedrus* and corresponding to the body's heart in the *Timaeus*.[6] Multiple early modern English writers on the topic acknowledge that 'some' people divide the soul, or just the highest part of the soul (the rational soul), into understanding and will. These writers also draw a distinction – although in different ways – between the will and appetite, with the will serving the soul and the appetite encompassing physical urges.[7] I take up the connection between will and soul at more length in Chapter 2; here, I just want to underline the usual placement of the will within the highest part of the soul – the part designed to guide and govern the self. Ultimately, Petruchio seeks to render Katharina an inanimate object, to drain her of her soul insofar as it encompasses her independent will by making her body 'passing empty' of food and energy – literally a weak and hollow vessel ready to receive his inspiration or direction (4.1.178). He appears to succeed. At the play's end, when Petruchio summons Katharina to demonstrate her obedience before the community at Bianca's wedding feast, Katharina's first words to Petruchio are 'What is your will, sir, that you send for me?' Then, when delivering the speech that Petruchio commands her to give, she calls that woman who is 'not obedient to [her husband's] honest will' a 'foul contending rebel / and graceless traitor' (5.2.104, 162–4).

And yet, at these moments when Katharina seems most puppet-like – as when, on Petruchio's absurd order, she throws her cap underfoot in front of the astonished wedding guests before lecturing the women present on the 'duty they do owe their lords and husbands' (135) – she is perhaps most beyond her puppeteer's control. Petruchio could have ventriloquized her final speech, in that it praises husbands so cloyingly and disparages women at such length for not believing their husbands to be their infinite superiors. But the excessiveness of this performance

⁵ William Shakespeare, *The Taming of the Shrew*, ed. David Bevington, 2.1.131–6. Subsequent references to *Shrew* cite this edition.

⁶ Rosalie Osmond, *Mutual Accusation*, 5.

⁷ See, for instance, John Woolton, *Immortalitie of the Soule*, 9; Simon Harward, *Discourse Concerning the Soule*, 12–13 (the folio page number appears erroneously as 31); Thomas Wright, *Passions of the Minde*, Ch. 8, 31–2, and John Davies, *Nosce Teipsum*, stanza 14.

of Petruchio's will (depending on its delivery, and in keeping with Katharina's sharp wit) undercuts its purported message about wifely subordination as natural. And this tactic of undercutting the message is beyond credible reproach, since any objection would force Petruchio and the men to admit that their own expectations sound over the top. Instead of truly becoming a puppet to her husband's will, Katharina arguably provides a puppet-like parody of Petruchio's notion of an ideal wife. Recent female directors of *Shrew* have certainly picked up on the possibility and potential of Katharina's disingenuous delivery of these final lines,[8] but the text itself hints that this rendering of the submission speech would not be so far-fetched even in Shakespeare's time. None of the husbands gathered at the wedding feast, for instance, has made the kind of self-sacrifices that Katharina praises so highly: not one of them has had to commit 'his body / To painful labor both by sea and land' or to 'watch the night in storms, the day in cold' in order to provide for his wife (152–4). Instead, they have all enjoyed a significant increase in finances, thanks to their new wives' dowries. If the implied mockery or criticism is lost on Petruchio and the wedding guests, it need not be lost on the audience.

Petruchio is not alone on the early modern stage in his desire to turn a woman into his puppet. In addition to the examples from *The Revenger's Tragedy* and *Bartholomew Fair* on which this chapter will focus, instances of men trying to puppet women both dead and alive turn up in a variety of Jacobean plays. In John Marston's *Sophonisba* (1606), for example, Masinissa makes Sophonisba's body a trophy to his honour after she has consumed poison to save him from his dilemma of either rendering his wife as a prize to the Roman general Scipio or breaking his oath to that general. Masinissa carefully orchestrates the public presentation of Sophonisba's body to Scipio: after a dramatic introduction he parades her body to the accompaniment of music (perhaps carried in a chair, as her body was borne offstage in the previous scene), and 'adorns' her corpse, most likely with the decoration he has just received from Scipio.[9] As he transfers his ornament to the dead Sophonisba, Masinissa fittingly declaims 'On thee, loved creature ... / Rest all *my* honour' (5.4.53–4, emphasis added), appropriating her body as an image of his own 'glory', 'virtue', and 'fame' – and procuring the status of 'Rome's very minion' as a result (42, 47). In *The Tempest* (1610), too, Prospero uses a number of spirits as puppets to do his bidding,[10] but perhaps he most resembles a puppet master when he demonstrates his ability to effortlessly remove Miranda from the conversation by casting her into a deep sleep and then reanimating her when it suits him, much as a puppeteer might cast aside his puppet and later take it up

---

8   See, for instance, Elizabeth Schafer, *Ms-Directing Shakespeare*, 65–8.

9   John Marston, *Sophonisba*, ed. Keith Sturgess, 5.4.44 sd, 54 sd.

10   For a thoughtful discussion of Prospero's spirit puppets, see Shershow, *Puppets*, 90–99. In Edmund Spenser's *The Faerie Queene*, I.i.38–I.ii.9, III.viii.4–10, the false Una that Archimago fashions to carry out his deceitful plans, and the sprites he summons to assist him, are immaterial or spirit puppets along the same lines, as is the false Florimell the witch creates.

again. The Tyrant in *The Lady's Tragedy*[11] (1611), a play I discuss at length in Chapter 3, tells the corpse of the Lady who, to escape his lust, committed suicide, 'I will possess thee' (4.3.116). Obsessed with her body – the 'house' to which 'the soul is but a tenant' (5.2.3) – he has it dressed, painted, and positioned ('Keep her up, / I'll have her swoon no more') to his liking (101–2).[12] And in Philip Massinger's *The Duke of Milan* (1621–1622?), the perfidious Francisco, disguised as a doctor, brags that through artifice he can convince the duke that the dead duchess lives again. As a puppeteer animates the lifeless puppet's body, Francisco claims that 'by a strange vapour, / Which I'll infuse into [the duchess's] mouth' he can 'create / A seeming breath' and 'make her veins run high too, / As if they had true motion'.[13] The duke's friend Pescara confidently hires him to do so.

The early modern habits of thought that view puppets as feminine and women as more likely than men to be puppet-like are inescapably misogynistic. 'Puppet' is a variant of 'poppet', a term of endearment, especially for 'a child or young woman', with the sense of 'darling' or 'pet'.[14] 'Poppet' – as well as similar words in other Romance and Germanic languages, such as the French 'poupée' – likely derives from the Latin 'puppa', meaning 'girl' or 'doll'.[15] Etymologically, then, femininity connects with the diminutive, the little – and relatedly, the inconsequential – in the word 'puppet'.[16] Puppets, of course, are material objects fashioned to be controlled by an external agent. They are inherently manipulable and their purpose is often to please the sight and to entertain. Apart from its denotative meaning, by the late sixteenth century the word 'puppet' held the derogatory connotation of 'a person,

---

[11]   I am convinced by the reasons Lisa Hopkins, *Female Hero*, 72, gives for using the title *The Lady's Tragedy* for Middleton's play, which has also been referred to as *The Second Maiden's Tragedy* and *The Maiden's Tragedy*. The following parenthetical references are to the performance text printed alongside the original text in Thomas Middleton, *The Lady's Tragedy*, ed. Gary Taylor and John Lavagnino.

[12]   Like *The Revenger's Tragedy*, this play is now widely accepted as Middleton's (both plays appear in Taylor and Lavagnino's recent *Thomas Middleton: The Collected Works*), and it presents interesting parallels to *Revenger's*.

[13]   Philip Massinger, *The Duke of Milan*, ed. Colin Gibson, 5.2.146–9.

[14]   *The Oxford English Dictionary Online (OED)*, 'poppet, n.', 1.

[15]   Ibid., a–d.

[16]   A search for the word 'puppet' in *Lexicons of Early Modern English* turns up results similar to the *OED* definitions that link the puppet with the feminine and the diminutive. An entry for 'Pupa' in the *Dictionarium Linguae Latinae et Anglicanae* (1587) reads 'A girle, a modder, a young wench: also a puppet like a girle'. An entry for 'pupo' in John Florio's *A World of Words* (1598) defines 'pupo' as 'a pigsneye, a sweet-hart, a prettie musse, a daintie mop, a playing babie, a puppet'. Florio's *Queen Anna's New World of Words* (1611) repeats this definition of 'pupo' and notes that 'Pupa', a 'babie or puppet like a girle', is 'Vsed also for a lasse or wench'. Edward Philips's *The New World of English Words* (1658) defines 'Mammet' as 'a puppet, from the Greek work Mamme, as it were a little Mother, or Nurse'. Shershow's helpful consideration in *Puppets* of the definitions of 'puppet' and related words first prompted me to consult the *OED* and *LEME* definitions.

esp. a woman, whose (esp. gaudy) dress or manner is thought to suggest a lack of substance or individuality'.[17] Besides the etymological roots of the word 'puppet', the puppet's need to be externally governed, its passivity, and its superficiality fit well with women's prescribed subordinate position to men in the patriarchal society of seventeenth-century England.[18] The hand puppet's hollowness without the puppeteer resonates with the early modern designation of woman as the 'weaker vessel' in relation to man – a designation enshrined in the King James Bible that gained proverbial status through its ubiquitous use for over a century.[19] Puppet and vessel both represent physical surfaces, empty unless filled with substance.

The puppet, in addition to its feminization and its resonance with the 'weaker vessel', also works as a basic metaphor for the relationship between body and soul. At this juncture, puppetry, as both performance and literary motif, provides a useful focal point to help illuminate the important connections between engagements of the body-soul dynamic and representations of women. Just as hand puppets might feature exaggerated physical features to catch the eye,[20] they can also foreground bluntly – which is not to say simplistically – questions about the relationship between inner and outer, spirit and matter, as these components made up the 'self'. As a hollow material body animated from within by the puppeteer, the hand puppet is most obviously analogous with a dualistic model of the self as consisting of two distinct components, a purely physical form animated by a separate, internal intelligence. In that the hand puppet permits the puppeteer to express his creative vision, the puppet is also comparable to the more Aristotelian notion of the body as a useful tool for the soul-as-artificer.[21] Both models find correspondence in humoural theory, which provides a language for recognizing the body's powerful influences on thought and feeling, and for controlling those influences through carefully regulated diet and activity.[22] The humoural system exemplifies the early

---

[17]   *OED*, 'puppet, n.', 3, emphasis added.

[18]   Male characters are puppeted onstage too, although when men are described or visually presented as puppet-like, the effect is usually to emphasize their effeminacy or deride them as undeserving social climbers, as Shershow, *Puppets*, 33, 72, 90, explains, culling examples from early modern theatre and literature. Shershow, 73, cites, for instance, satirical comparisons of 'the specter of social mobility' with puppets, or 'the performing object', in Marston, Chapman, and Middleton; Falstaff's 'analogy between the diminutive and the artificial' in his descriptions of his page, 76–7; and the 'puppetlike gull' Sir Politic Would-Be, who is mocked as a 'rare motion' when found hiding in a tortoise shell, 88.

[19]   See Anthony Fletcher, *Gender, Sex and Subordination*, 60–61, on the 'common usage' of the term 'weaker vessel' to designate women.

[20]   Such as, for instance, the puppets featured in Antoni Cimolino's 2009 direction of *Bartholomew Fair* in Stratford, Ontario.

[21]   See Osmond, *Mutual Accusation*, 6–7, 14–15, for a discussion of Aristotle's concept of the body as an instrument for the soul.

[22]   For more on the measure of control over one's body and temperament that the language of humoural theory enabled, see Michael Schoenfeldt, *Bodies and Selves*, especially 11–13, 20–23. Further examples of the body as under the soul's control or

modern understanding of the body as a useful tool, but one that requires proper surveillance and governance. Women's bodies required the most surveillance and governance – humoural theory helped naturalize the construction of women as less in control of their own bodies than men were, and, as a result, more vulnerable to unruly passions, which the body was believed to generate.[23] Men, who were supposedly not as prone to bodily influence, were considered more able to exercise reason, a faculty of the soul, and theological ideas that God ordained the soul to govern the body, and man to govern woman, were naturalized through cross-reference or analogy.[24]

The puppet onstage, I argue, especially when that puppet represents an actual woman, must be interpreted in light of this network of associations that connected femininity, materiality, the body, and emotion and placed them below masculinity, immateriality, the soul, and reason. These cultural resonances make the puppet a particularly potent metaphor for the use of a woman as a man's mere instrument to achieve his own ends, whether the goal be vengeance or social advancement. Indeed, because of these deeper associations, onstage allusions to puppetry render this treatment of women even more violent, aggressive, and dismissive of the complexity of female subjectivity than initially appears. The attempt to 'puppet' a woman, in other words, conveys a complete denial of a complex subjectivity rooted at once in body and spirit. Puppetry is an emptying out of her soul, a reduction and simplification that equates her with her body and attempts to ensoul that body with the puppeteer's self-serving agenda. Katharine Eisaman Maus identifies an early modern 'sense of discrepancy' between 'socially

---

instruction include the eighth emblem in book 5 of Francis Quarles's *Emblemes*, which shows a skeleton (representing the body) waiting, in boredom, for the soul within its ribcage to finish praying, and George Herbert's 'Church Monuments', in which the speaker directs his 'flesh' to 'learn' amidst entombed ashes 'thy stem / And true descent' while the speaker's soul is praying.

[23] Gail Kern Paster, *Body Embarrassed*, 25, discusses how 'discourse about the female body' in texts, including plays, 'Renaissance medical texts, iconography, and the proverbs of oral culture ... [i]nscribes women as leaky vessels by isolating one element of the female body's material expressiveness – its production of fluids – as excessive, hence either disturbing or shameful'. The 'issue is women's bodily self-control or, more precisely, the representation of a particular kind of uncontrol as a function of gender'. While Paster is not interested in how this inscription might affect concepts of women's souls, Schoenfeldt's convincing argument in *Bodies and Selves* that physiological experience and psychological inwardness are 'fully imbricated', with Galenic medicine providing a discourse that articulated 'human emotion in corporeal terms' (1, 6–11), would suggest that the construction of women as having no control over their bodies would translate to a corresponding lack of control over their spiritual states. Indeed, Gwynne Kennedy, in *Just Anger*, 6–8, gathers persuasive evidence that women were thought to be more prone to unruly emotions because of their supposedly weaker minds, and likely to express inferior or more childish and less 'legitimate' forms of emotion (namely anger) than men because of their 'inferior' physical constitution.

[24] See Kennedy, *Just Anger*, 1–2, 4, and Osmond, *Mutual Accusation*, 157–60.

visible' exteriors and 'invisible personal' interiors, a discrepancy that influenced concepts of subjectivity reflected in Renaissance drama and poetry.[25] The notion of inner 'disposition' and outer 'appearance' could be employed, she explains, for self-protection, as one could conform outwardly to the government-imposed religion, for instance, while concealing within one's real beliefs.[26] In some cases, a 'highly developed sense of personal inwardness' is 'intrinsic' to challenges to authority, and while selves were considered 'obscure' and 'hidden', they were also considered 'capable of being made fully manifest',[27] as the violent plucking out of a traitor's heart on the scaffold gruesomely dramatizes.[28] With similar violence, the onstage act of puppeting a woman effaces in her the kind of inwardness Maus and Elizabeth Hanson see as linked to rebelliousness by assuming, in its place, an inherent emptiness to be filled. The male character alluded to as the puppeteer of a female character takes to the extreme the cultural association of masculinity with superior reasoning ability and a closer proximity to the divine by assuming an almost god-like role, fashioning, in a sense, a woman that suits him and delighting in controlling her – that is, in constituting her inner animating force. As I will discuss further on, Vindice and Littlewit are both artist figures who express delight – absolute glee in Vindice's case – in the artistic presentation of their respective female puppets. But the puppetry in both *The Revenger's Tragedy* and *Bartholomew Fair* eventually (and perhaps paradoxically) works to expose the grave error of Vindice and the absurdity of Littlewit taking on this role of puppet master in relation to women.

Indeed, while the puppet as metaphor seems a straightforward illustration of the conventional, gendered divide between body and soul, animated and animator, in performance the puppet does not always bear out these neat divisions. Instead, it holds potential to radically subvert them. Puppets appearing alongside actors onstage – whether the puppeted skull (and eventually the entire skeleton) of Gloriana in *The Revenger's Tragedy*, or Leatherhead's hand puppets in *Bartholomew Fair* – can quickly take on personalities (or perhaps an aura, in Gloriana's case) all their own. Any clean distinction between animated and animator, dull material and immaterial force becomes confused when the puppets seem to have a distinct influence over the puppeteer and a predominant place in the audience's attention.[29] As much as the puppeteer might emphasize absolute control

---

[25]   Katharine Eisaman Maus, *Inwardness and Theatre*, 12–13.

[26]   Ibid., 18–24.

[27]   Ibid., 70, 28–9. For more on the 'alliance between inwardness and agency in the service of self-interest' and on inwardness as the 'subversive or even demonic' ability to 'operate secretly beyond the constraints of constituted authority', see Elizabeth Hanson, *Discovering the Subject*, especially 16–18.

[28]   Hanson, *Discovering the Subject*, 1.

[29]   Puppets indeed held the potential to be 'show-stealers', as Ejner J. Jensen's survey of reviews of Terry Hands's 1969 production of *Bartholomew Fair* at the Aldwych, in Jensen, *Ben Jonson's Comedies*, 49, indicates. Despite several reviewers' objections to various

over the puppet, just as Petruchio's figurative puppet, Katharina, moves beyond his intentions while seeming to execute his orders, puppets have a tendency to exceed authorial intention. This sometimes-eerie tendency raises the possibility that the material might have a spirit and agenda of its own apart from the animation of the puppeteer (and even the playwright). The puppet, in other words, reverses the usual connection, identified by Maus and Hanson, between inwardness, mystery, and rebelliousness. While the puppet's interior is no secret, its exterior captivates the imagination and carries potential to signify something other than its governing interior intends. Before discussing the significance of specific examples to stage representations of women, I want to briefly suggest two sources of the puppet's defiant and even threatening nature: its frequent parodic role in early modern puppet shows belonging to 'low' or vulgar entertainment, and its similarity to – especially for Puritan anti-theatricalists – an idol.

Early modern puppet shows were not performances one would attend for moral edification or the presentation of a serious narrative – or even a coherent or logical narrative at that. Rather, they were often hilarious burlesques of biblical, historical, mythical, and literary narratives that 'flourished', as George Speaight informs us, in 'the sub-world of popular entertainment'. Motions were performed 'in temporary booths or in hired rooms at fairs, at inns, and on busy street corners'.[30] Speaight describes the 'Elizabethan motion' as 'a robust, unsophisticated entertainment … with no attempt at historical accuracy, and spiced with topical allusions'.[31] Sometimes 'subjects were … borrowed from popular plays in the human theatre', and 'heroes from the history of all ages might be ridiculously jumbled together in a slapstick buffoonery' with 'the story … conveyed in the crudest of jog-trot verse'.[32] An example showing the flavour of the giddy, 'incongruous' mixture of 'topical allusion' with biblical, historical, and literary narratives that Speaight cites is 'when the notorious brothels of Sodom and Gomorrah were seen to be

---

aspects of the production, the puppet show was praised as 'the best part of the play' and the point at which the evening 'came to life', the puppets being 'more alive and human than the characters in the play'. For a more general discussion of how the categories of 'subject' and 'object' – which the puppeteer and puppet fit into – are unstable in Renaissance England, and how subjectivity can both be constituted through objects and collapse into objects, see Margreta De Grazia et al. (eds), *Subject and Object in Renaissance Culture*.

[30] Speaight, *English Puppet Theatre*, 63, 60. Speaight, 60–62, establishes 'five pitches in London at which puppet shows were given' from 'the mass of vague contemporary allusions', but reminds us that 'the London performances were, however, comparatively unimportant for the puppet showmen, and the majority of these made their living by touring the country'. See also Shershow, *Puppets*, 45 and n. 1, for descriptions of the venues and surrounding atmosphere of puppet performances and for further references.

[31] Speaight, *English Puppet Theatre*, 17.

[32] Ibid., 64. Speaight gives several examples from his extensive research into the history of the English puppet theatre to support these assertions. See his Ch. IV, 'Puppets in England: From Chaucer to Cromwell', 52–72.

demolished by a crowd of Elizabethan apprentices'.[33] Leatherhead mentions this Sodom and Gomorrah action when reminiscing, in *Bartholomew Fair*, about the past motions he has performed, and Speaight singles out Jonson's play as a particularly illuminating source on what early modern English puppet shows were like.[34]

If Jonson's puppet show of 'Hero and Leander' in *Bartholomew Fair* indicates any regular features of puppet theatre, then the mere sight of a puppet poised to perform would undoubtedly excite in an audience expectations of parody; rebelliousness (the puppets repeatedly interrupt and beat their puppet master); and an overall sense of bursting out of all bounds (the puppets cannot refrain from beating one another up at the slightest provocation, their vulgar behaviour and language observe no limits, and limits also do not apply to what material can be blended together and burlesqued in their play). Puppet shows certainly took irreverent liberties with esteemed narratives by abandoning (if not outright mocking) whatever ideals, moral lessons, or tragedies could be found in the stories they adapted in favour of 'a more familiar strain for our people'.[35] They also included very physical, bawdy comedy. In this 'debasing' process, which involved the audience by inciting their laughter, puppets function as a kind of social levelling force. Overall, the puppet performing in fairs, at bridges, and on busy street corners was well known for its traditionally parodic role, and when transferred to the human stage, the puppet's connection to parody and irreverence contributes to its potential to unsettle the very dichotomies it at first seems to illustrate.

The puppet's strong connections to the profane, however, should not completely obscure its connections to the spiritual. Before the Reformation, puppets played a role in liturgical drama, perhaps even portraying the Passion, the visit of the three Marys to Christ's tomb, and the Resurrection, and they were probably 'occasionally employed in the open-air miracle plays that succeeded the church performances'.[36] The word 'marionette' (little Mary) may have 'referred originally to the sculpted figures of the Virgin' in crèches or nativity scenes.[37] Protestant denunciation of

---

[33]   Ibid., 64.

[34]   Ibid., 57–60.

[35]   Ben Jonson, *Bartholomew Fair*, ed. Helen Ostovich, 5.3.96. All references to the play cite this edition.

[36]   Victoria Nelson, *Secret Life of Puppets*, 49; Shershow, *Puppets*, 40; Speaight, *English Puppet Theatre*, 53–4. The evidence Speaight cites in support of marionettes in mystery plays consists of the mayor of Chester's disapproving reference, in 1599, to 'god on strings' and a 'stage direction in a Cornish mystery of 1611' that 'calls for "every degree of devils of leather and spirits on cords"'.

[37]   Shershow, *Puppets*, 40. Jonas Barish, '*Bartholomew Fair* and Its Puppets', 14, n. 21, notes E.K. Chambers's earlier suggestion that 'the use of puppets' to portray the nativity is a practice that 'survives in the Christmas *crèche*'. Shershow, *Puppets*, 26–7, also draws attention to the word 'mammet', a common early modern English word for puppet, which, according to *OED* 1.a, c, refers to 'a false god', 'an image of a false god', or 'an idol', and was derogatory 'in Protestant usage' for 'an image of Christ or of a saint, etc., as used in Roman Catholic practice'.

Catholicism's ritualistic use of material objects in worship as superstitious and idolatrous often compares Catholic ritual itself to the performance of puppetry.[38] Without retracing the well-documented invocation of the puppet as a prime symbol of idolatry, especially in anti-Catholic rhetoric (which, as Zeal-of-the-land Busy shows us, merges seamlessly with anti-theatrical rhetoric),[39] I simply want to underline the point that, although not relics or ritualistic objects themselves in Catholic practice, puppets became associated with the idea – so inimical to Protestant belief – of material not animated by, or the mere shell of, a governing soul, but itself imbued with spirit or having potent spiritual significance.[40]

In performance the puppet can really come to life, in a sense, as material infused with spirit somehow beyond the movements generated by the puppeteer's hand and exuding parody that escapes the puppeteer's interpretations. In performance, puppets both emphatically foreground the material and unsettle the dominant construction of spirit or soul in opposition to material. This unsettling, I posit, has repercussions for the representation of women, who were aligned with the material and the body in opposition to men, aligned with the soul, and who became puppets onstage far more often than did male characters.[41] In what follows, I examine two vastly different instances of puppetry onstage – Vindice's gruesome

---

[38] Shershow, *Puppets*, 38–9, 76–81, supplies two representative early modern examples of the Catholic Eucharistic Host being likened to a kind of deceiving puppet.

[39] Refer especially to Shershow, *Puppets*, 22–42. See also Susan Zimmerman, *Early Modern Corpse*, 26–7, and Chs 2 and 3 on 'the corpse as idol'; Thomas Rist, *Revenge Tragedy*, 3–26, on similarities between the performance of Catholic funerary ritual and theatrical performance of revenge tragedy; Melinda Gough, 'Jonson's Siren Stage', 69, 71, 76, for a discussion of the temptress in anti-theatrical writings and epic romance as a figure associated with idolatry and parodied by the puppet; and Nelson, *Secret Life of Puppets*, 30–31, 42–3, on connections between puppets and idols apart from anti-theatrical or anti-Catholic rhetoric.

[40] The Protestant invocation of the idol (and puppet-as-idol) as a sign of the mistaken belief or superstition that certain material objects held spiritual properties could, instead of foregrounding the emptiness or deadness of the material, paradoxically invest the idol with more sinister magical properties. In that the idol lured one away from true spiritual connection with God, it could be seen as a tool of the devil, as Milton makes clear in the Argument of book I of *Paradise Lost*, in which hell's 'chief leaders' are 'named, according to the idols known afterwards in Canaan and the countries adjoining'. For a discussion of 'image magic' and the belief that puppets were used as demonic tools in witchcraft, refer to Shershow, *Puppets*, 33–7.

[41] *The Revenger's Tragedy* presents the less common case of a male character's body being physically puppeted when Vindice and Hippolito dress up the Duke's corpse as Piato (Vindice's persona when disguised) and position it to appear as if it were alive and slouched over in a drunken stupor. This puppeting of the Duke, however, is a spontaneous act intended to deceive Lussurioso, who has ordered the brothers to murder Piato before his eyes, whereas Vindice's puppeting of Gloriana is an obsessive and long-drawn-out practice. She has been dead for nine years, and Hippolito's comment that Vindice is 'still sighing o'er Death's vizard' suggests that he has not just recently unearthed her remains (1.1.50).

and silent puppetry of Gloriana's skull and Leatherhead's boisterous and hilarious booth puppetry – to suggest that in these plays, often noted for their pronounced misogyny, puppetry significantly troubles the predominant system of thought that subordinated the material, emotional, and feminine to the spiritual, rational, and masculine.

Gloriana's Grin: Material Disrupting Meaning in *The Revenger's Tragedy*

> There is some hidden power in these dead things
> That calls my flesh into'em.
>
> – Amintor in *The Maid's Tragedy* (5.3.181–2)

Vindice turns the bare skull – the body part Helkiah Crooke would later designate as the 'mansion house' of 'the soule'[42] – and, in act 3, possibly the skeletal body of the murdered lady once betrothed to him, into his puppet, a mere hollow tool he strategically employs to achieve his own ends. He 'fashion[s]' this puppet himself by dressing it *'up in tires'*[43] and, manipulating its physical movements, he both interprets its meaning to Hippolito and the audience[44] and animates it with his personal desire for revenge against the Duke (who poisoned Gloriana after failing to seduce her, and whom Vindice also blames for the death of his father).[45] Vindice appears as the dead Gloriana's puppet master, rather than as her bereaved fiancé. He takes intense pleasure in the artistic set-up of his revenge against the Duke, and he delights in orchestrating events to serve poetic justice according to his own

---

[42] Helkiah Crooke, *Mikrokosmographia*, book 1, Ch. 4, 10.

[43] Thomas Middleton, *The Revenger's Tragedy*, ed. Brian Gibbons, 3.5.42 sd, 99. Subsequent references to the play cite this edition.

[44] Puppet shows often featured an interpreter. In *Bartholomew Fair* Leatherhead is both puppet master and interpreter as he explains and clarifies the puppets' lines for Cokes. Speaight, *English Puppet Theatre*, 67, discusses the possible origin and role of the puppet 'interpreter': 'some puppet shows were brought by foreigners, Italians or French, who could not speak English, and so hired a native to stand outside the booth to translate, or interpret, what was being said. But, quite apart from any difficulty of language, the interpreter seems to have been needed to translate the puppets' speeches even when they spoke in English', likely because of efforts to 'give a distinctive tone to the puppets' speech'. Speaight lists several contemporary references to puppet interpreters and to the strangeness of puppets' voices.

[45] I agree here with Kathryn R. Finin, '"Wild Justice" and the Female Body', par. 25, who claims that 'critics (mis)led by Vindice have pointed to Gloriana's participation as an example of female agency, yet to call this her revenge further elides the violence enacted upon her mutilated corpse. Despite the rhetorical sleight of hand through which Vindice aligns Gloriana's interests with his own, his description of her "ravishment" as "delectable" and "rare" directs our attention to the self-interested nature of his representation'.

script – a script, as Kathryn R. Finin puts it aptly, that is 'primarily concerned with the aesthetics rather than the ethics of revenge'.[46]

Beyond enabling the 'aesthetically perfect' surprise that Vindice reserves for his enemy,[47] a poisonous kiss from the very body the Duke himself poisoned for first refusing his lust, Vindice's puppet master role also fits with his meta-theatrical attitude. More than once, Vindice draws attention to stage practice. Appalled by the depravity of the Duke's son Lussurioso, he expresses 'wonder' that 'such a fellow, impudent and wicked, / Should not be cloven as he stood', and asks 'Is there no thunder left, or is't kept up / In stock for heavier vengeance?' The sound effect of thunder answers Vindice on cue – 'There it goes!' (4.2.193–8). For Jonathan Dollimore, 'here the traditional invocation to heaven becomes a kind of public stage-prompt' and 'the conception of a heavenly, retributive justice is being reduced to a parody of stage effects'.[48] With reference to similar moments (such as Vindice's comments that 'When the bad bleeds, then is the tragedy good' [3.5.199], or, upon the sound of thunder at the murder of the newly installed Duke Lussurioso, 'Mark; thunder! Dost know thy cue'? [5.3.43–4]), Dollimore notes that Vindice is 'invested with a theatrical sense resembling the dramatist's own'.[49] When Vindice assumes the 'identity' of dramatist, the effect is to 'shatter' the 'dramatic illusion' just when it 'needs to be strongest' if 'the providential references are to convince'.[50] Vindice's role of puppet master echoes the role of dramatist he assumes in both the meta-theatrical sense and in the play itself with his glee at how well 'suited' his revenge is to the Duke's crimes (3.5.28–32). More important, Vindice's puppetry of Gloriana reflects the hollowing-out effect that his dramatist attitude has on traditional notions of divine retribution. In the same way that his allusions to stage convention deny thunder any heavenly power, his callous use of Gloriana's remains as 'a thing' and stage 'property' to assist in his plot denies her bones a sacrosanct status, presenting them instead as barren of any spiritual significance.

Vindice's complete irreverence for Gloriana's skull has led Thomas Rist to set *The Revenger's Tragedy* apart from other early modern revenge tragedies that, as Rist discusses, invest material with spiritual significance by placing importance on performative ritual practices in remembrance of the dead.[51] The ghosts that often turn up in this genre, worried about being forgotten, suggest that 'remembrance *effects* the dead'.[52] The solemn portrayal of ritual commemoration of the dead, the appearance of ghosts anxious about the integrity of their corpses, and even the necessarily physical representations of ghosts onstage resonate with Catholic

---

[46] Finin, '"Wild Justice" and the Female Body', par. 3.

[47] Ibid., par. 21.

[48] Jonathan Dollimore, *Radical Tragedy*, 140.

[49] Ibid.

[50] Ibid.

[51] Rist, *Revenge Tragedy*, 4, 8, 14, 17, 100–105.

[52] Ibid., 14.

emphasis on the interpenetration of spirit and matter.[53] Protestant thinkers, as Susan Zimmerman summarizes, viewed 'the Catholic system of worship' as 'hypostatis[ing] the body, thereby privileging the material principle over that of the spiritual'. To 'counteract the materiality of Catholicism' they 'needed to draw sharper distinctions between the material and the spiritual'.[54] Rist finds that *The Revenger's Tragedy* has more affinity with reformist ideas in that it persistently demystifies and 'mocks remembrances of the dead' as ineffective, as 'bare and empty' as Gloriana's bones, her skull 'a plaything rather than a thing of honour', and the dead powerless against the abuses of the living.[55]

But Gloriana's appearance as Vindice's 'plaything' – literally, his puppet, a performative object with the potential of materially signifying meaning to the audience beyond or contradictory to the puppeteer's voiced intentions – is precisely what should alert us to the important distinction between the effect Gloriana might have on the audience and Vindice's treatment and interpretation of her. In Gloriana, the uncanny, intermediary status of the puppet, with its traditional spiritual associations despite its blatant materiality, together with its capacity to confuse the lines between animated and animator, overlaps with the intermediary status of the human corpse. The corpse occupied a doubly liminal position between death and burial and, in its state of decomposition, between flesh and dust. A popular though unorthodox belief held that the soul might linger near its corpse prior to interment and perhaps even longer.[56] This notion about some form of continuing tie between soul and body after death, a connection between the 'sanctity of the grave' and the 'repose of the soul', is further evidenced in the intense controversy over human dissection.[57] Both Catholics and Protestants

---

[53]   See Peter Stallybrass, 'Hauntings: The Materiality of Memory', for a fascinating discussion of the materiality of stage ghosts, which were often represented bearing the marks of their bodily deaths, and for a consideration of the material connection between the living and the dead that adhered through passed-down belongings.

[54]   Zimmerman, *Early Modern Corpse*, 25, 28. Zimmerman, 45–6, explains that although 'in early modern England, the categorical distinctions of Cartesian philosophy had not yet come to dominate any sphere of intellectual life, including that of religion … Protestant iconoclasm shifted discursive emphasis from the interdependence of body and soul to the priority of the spirit, and in so doing established a prototypical paradigm for mind/body duality. Nonetheless, the development of the reformist movement was hardly linear or univocal, so that the concepts and/or symbolic matrices of the old and new religions often fused in ways that defied categorical description'.

[55]   Rist, *Revenge Tragedy*, 98–106.

[56]   David Cressy, *Birth, Marriage, and Death*, 398, notes that 'some people believed that the soul still lingered in the vicinity of the body during the first thirty days after burial, a liminal situation requiring great ritual caution'. Similarly, 'for people who believed that the soul or spirit was not fully detached, and might in some way hover or linger during that liminal interval between death and interment, the experience of watching [the body prior to burial] could be full of terrors' (428).

[57]   Ruth Richardson, *Death, Dissection and the Destitute*, 75–6, discusses 'popular hostility to dissection' as constituting 'a gross assault upon the integrity and identity of

widely believed in the eventual resurrection of the body and its reunion with the soul at the last judgement.[58] This belief meant that the body was not irrelevant after death; it was an essential component of the immortal self and, as such, merited respect and safekeeping in a proper grave.[59] In the overflowing churchyards of early modern England, of course, old graves were frequently disturbed, as bones were inevitably unearthed in the preparation of new graves. The common practice of collecting these loose bones into charnel-houses to make room for new churchyard tenants meant that the prospect of disinterred bones, in itself, would not be especially disturbing to a seventeenth-century audience.[60] Vindice's employment of Gloriana's skull, however, is not comparable to the inadvertent uncovering of random bones that were consequently bequeathed to the shelter of the charnel house. Vindice targets Gloriana's body and intentionally keeps it from its grave, prolonging her liminal status as an unburied corpse. If Vindice exhibits no qualms in puppeting what he sees as an empty 'shell of Death', the audience need not follow his lead. In fact, the discrepancy between the possibility that Gloriana's bones, on some level, remain of interest to her departed spirit and Vindice's callous and even bitter objectification of her remains can create a distinct atmosphere of discomfort. Several critics signal awareness of this discomfort when they speak about Vindice as desecrating, violating, or prostituting Gloriana's bones.[61]

I want to suggest that a challenge to Vindice's misogynistic attitude is bound up in the challenge that Gloriana's stage presence poses to notions of the

---

the body *and* upon the repose of the soul'. See also Clare Gittings, *Death, Burial, and the Individual*, 74–5, and Zimmerman, *Early Modern Corpse*, 132–4.

[58]   Cressy, *Birth, Marriage, and Death*, 387.

[59]   Ibid., 389, notes that 'once buried, a body could not be exhumed without official permission'. A body committed to the grave 'belonged to no one. It lay, now, in God's freehold, and was subject to ecclesiastical cognizance if removed or abused'. Cressy explains that 'though materially dead', bodies 'deserved reverential treatment' as former 'vessels of the soul' that were 'destined to rise again'. He cites Anthony Sparrow's illuminating description later in the century (1668) of the corpse 'not as a lost and perished carcase, but as having in it a seed of eternity'. Gittings, *Death, Burial, and the Individual*, 60, suggests that 'no doubt some people, particularly among the uneducated, held extremely literal interpretations of the resurrection, making the correct burial of dead bodies a matter of vital importance in their eschatological scheme. In popular belief, a Christian funeral was held to assist the passage of the soul to the hereafter. Without these rites, it was felt, the soul might "walk"'.

[60]   For details on the over-crowding of churchyards and the need for 'bonehouses', see Gittings, *Death, Burial, and the Individual*, 149–50, and Cressy, *Birth, Marriage, and Death*, 380.

[61]   To cite a few examples, Finin, '"Wild Justice" and the Female Body', pars 24–5, discusses the 'sexual violence' enacted upon Gloriana's remains and how Vindice's 'restoring the female body ... restores its rapable possibilities'; Steven Mullaney, 'Mourning and Misogyny', 258, describes Gloriana as a 'representation of sovereign sexuality fully mastered and fully violated'; and Zimmerman, *Early Modern Corpse*, 135, 141, also describes the skeleton as 'violated' and Vindice as a 'sacrilegious puppeteer'.

material as the binary opposite of the spiritual, inherently empty of any intangible influence. Despite most of its characters' clearly expressed misogyny, a few critics have suggested that *The Revenger's Tragedy* in some ways provides what Steven Mullaney calls 'a critical examination of the tradition' of 'stage misogyny'.[62] Mullaney, Zimmerman, and Finin, for instance, notice that Vindice himself becomes the epitome of his own negative view of women, Mullaney referring to how 'Vindice ends the play as the leaky vessel he thought to distinguish himself from' by 'dribbling away his secret' when, unsolicited, he confesses to murder only because he cannot resist vanity – he needs to brag about how wittily he executed his plot.[63] Even before the play exposes Vindice's hypocrisy in this way, Gloriana presents him, as we shall see, with an unheeded warning of his downfall. Lynette McGrath records how 'the masculine soul, not the female body, was identified in the early modern period with the individual self, the mind, or the spirit', and finds that since women, 'especially in Puritan ideology', were 'ever more essentialized in physical terms', they found ways to 'invest some sense of self in their physicality'.[64] The tendency to align subjectivity and intelligence with physicality and the body that McGrath discovers in women's writing combats the denial of complex female subjectivity otherwise inherent in the misogynistic identification of woman as body. This challenge turns not on a counter-emphasis on woman as soul (which, as we know, only creates the problematic polarization of women into categories of either chaste maid or evil whore), but on the rejection of the body-soul, material-immaterial divide altogether. Applying McGrath's insight to Gloriana would be a stretch, and I certainly do not intend to claim any subjectivity or intelligence for Gloriana's skull. But this strategy McGrath identifies in women's writing holds relevance, I think, for the effect of Gloriana's stage presence in that, by blurring the neat lines of the material-immaterial divide in a different way, Gloriana poses an eerie threat or warning to those who, like Vindice, both discursively link women to the material and devalue the material as void of and inferior to the spiritual.

Vindice's soliloquies to Gloriana's skull, which might be expected to suggest an immaterial bond to Gloriana that has outlasted death, really only reveal how Vindice identifies Gloriana 'as body' both before and after her death, and serve to interpret her in these terms to the audience, much as an interpreter explains the puppets to the audience of a motion. Alluding to the memento mori tradition, Vindice introduces (and possessively objectifies) Gloriana as 'My

---

[62]   Mullaney, 'Mourning and Misogyny', 259.

[63]   Ibid.; Zimmerman, 'Marginal Man', 174; Finin, '"Wild Justice" and the Female Body', par. 13. Karin S. Coddon, 'Necrophilia and *The Revenger's Tragedy*', 71, 75, argues that 'necrophilia in *The Revenger's Tragedy* ... parod[ies]' and 'interrogate[s] contemporary, increasingly scientist notions of the body' which tended to irrationalize the female body and converge with 'means' to control it. Coddon, 76, also points out that since 'the skull is gendered only because we are told so', it exposes the contrivance of gender categories.

[64]   Lynette McGrath, *Subjectivity and Women's Poetry*, 29, 31.

study's ornament' (1.1.15). Beyond serving as a sombre moral reminder of the eventual decay of all things earthly, however, the memento mori should direct contemplation to the spiritual and the afterlife – an aspect that Vindice completely overlooks. Besides a brief mention of how the living Gloriana's eyes were 'heaven-pointed' and a vague reference to Gloriana's 'purer part', which 'would not consent' to the Duke's lust, Vindice never elaborates upon or again refers to Gloriana's soul or virtues (1.1.19, 33). Instead, he expresses disgust at the 'ragged imperfections' or 'unsightly rings' of her eye-sockets, juxtaposing them with a memory of her living 'face / So far beyond the artificial shine / Of any woman's bought complexion' (18–22). This memory, however, immediately slides from expressing admiration at Gloriana's superior natural beauty to associating it with carnal temptation and deception: her beauty could have caused 'the uprightest man' to sin just 'with looking after her', and 'she was able to ha' made a usurer's son / Melt all his patrimony in a kiss' (23–9). Tellingly, Vindice refers to the living Gloriana as 'Thee when thou wert apparelled in thy flesh' (31), a description that emphasizes a passive physicality (her body is mere decoration or garment) and that could just as easily apply to a corpse, as the later appearance onstage of the fully fleshed corpse of Antonio's wife reminds us. Of course, the soul could also be described as wearing a garment of flesh, but since Vindice is directly addressing Gloriana's skull here, he seems to leave the soul out of the equation entirely. The possibility that he implicitly addresses Gloriana's soul vanishes as Vindice continues his address: 'Advance thee, oh thou terror to fat folks / To have their costly three-piled flesh worn off / As bare as this' (45–7). Not only is he clearly referring to the skull alone here, but with the words 'advance thee' we could imagine him advancing towards the audience and thrusting the skull, his puppet, forward – but as grim spectacle and macabre joke instead of as revered relic of his murdered beloved.

Vindice does not discount the existence of souls altogether. To list a few instances, he speaks of having to 'blister my soul' (2.2.36), of his father's 'smothered' 'spirit' (1.2.124), and of 'torturing' the Duke's 'soul' (3.5.20). But he only refers explicitly to women's souls when their status affects his own male honour. He threatens his mother, Gratiana, with daggers for bending to the persuasions of a stranger (really Vindice disguised) and thereby consenting to pressure her daughter, Castiza, to offer her body to the lust of the Duke's son Lussurioso in the hope of material gain. When Gratiana weeps out the repentance she has very much been forced to express, Vindice is content to take it as 'a sweet shower, it does much good; / The fruitful grounds and meadows of her soul / Has been long dry' (4.4.47–9). He proposes to his brother to 'now' kiss her and 'marry her to our souls, wherein's no lust, / And honourably love her' (57–9). Indeed, the brothers can 'honourably' love Gratiana again, now that they have terrorizingly dealt with the threat to their honour that she was posing, and Vindice, positioning himself as knowing judge of her soul, has decided that it has been renewed and a 'foul name' – for the family as much as for Gratiana – avoided. Vindice goes on to reflect bitterly on what Castiza would have become had Gratiana succeeded,

> The duke's son's great concubine!
> A drab of state, a cloth o' silver slut,
> To have her train borne up and her soul
> Trail i' the dirt: great! (71–4)

These strong terms of contempt to describe a completely groundless, imagined version of his sister frame a reference to her soul that presents its hypothetical fall more as an almost-visible public embarrassment (like the exposure and dirtying of a private undergarment) than as a personal moral crisis for Castiza.

Vindice's conventional treatment of the female soul's virtue as inextricable from the honour or chastity of the body echoes in Antonio's interpretation of his wife's suicide: 'She, her honour forced, / Deemed it a nobler dowry for her name / To die with poison than to live with shame' (1.4.46–8). In other words, no part of her could escape the 'shame' of her body's rape except through death. The relentless correlation between the honour of body and soul while the woman is living,[65] however, gives neither man pause before subjecting her dead body to precisely the kind of dishonour that she died avoiding (Gloriana) or trying to forget (Antonio's wife). Antonio's wife kills herself after the traumatic experience of being 'harried' and having 'her honour forced' at a public event 'amidst a throng of pandars' (43–6), only to have her body again displayed before a 'throng' of men, this time exposed by her husband (perhaps with the dramatic flourish of a suddenly opened curtain) to '*certain lords*', Piero, and Hippolito (0 sd). As the Duke's younger son uses her body to serve his lust, Antonio appropriates his wife's body to serve and advance his own honour. He ends the sombre scene expressing 'joy' that 'being an old man I'd a wife so chaste' (75–8), and despite repeated references to how her death brings renown to her 'name' (47, 50, 70–71), we never do find out what her name is; we know her only as Antonio's wife, and as her name is subsumed by her husband, so is her honour.

I have digressed to consider briefly Antonio's 'reveal' because the play sets up thematically a double parallel between Antonio's treatment of his wife's corpse and her rapist's treatment of her living body on one side, and Vindice's treatment of what remains of Gloriana's corpse and the Duke's treatment of Gloriana's body on the other. The effect of these parallels is to invite criticism, or, at the very least, questioning of the treatment not just of women's bodies, but of their dead bodies, as mere material – that is, material understood in opposition to spiritual significance.

Vindice mirrors the Duke, who attempted to prostitute Gloriana to his lust and murdered her for resisting, by prostituting the physical remnants of Gloriana to

---

[65]   Lussurioso makes this correlation explicit when hiring Vindice (disguised as Piato) to convince Vindice's own sister to offer herself to Lussurioso's lust. He instructs Vindice: 'Enter upon the portion of her soul, / Her honour, which she calls her chastity, / And bring it into expense' (1.3.115–17). Here, 'chastity' or bodily honour is the 'portion' or dowry of Castiza's soul; Lussurioso couches the correlation between body and soul in financial terms.

his lust for revenge against the Duke. After dying to keep her body intact from the Duke's touch, Gloriana's skull-face is smeared with the very poison that killed her and subjected to the invasive, 'slobbering' tongue of her murderer (3.5.163).[66] The very act of puppeting Gloriana's skull, and possibly her skeleton – if, taking a cue from Vindice, who labels her 'the bony lady' (120), we are to imagine a skeleton beneath her costume – potentially suggests that Vindice's manipulation of Gloriana's remains has its own disturbingly sexual component. Is Vindice's hand up Gloriana's skirts in order to support and move her in a way not obvious to the Duke? This possibility might put us in mind of the later sexually charged image of De Flores 'thrust[ing]' his fingers into the 'sockets' of Beatrice-Joanna's glove in *The Changeling*[67] – a manipulation of material once attached to her that makes De Flores's violent lust for Beatrice-Joanna startlingly clear. And even if Vindice's method of puppetry does not involve a hand concealed in Gloriana's garments, does he move her in any way, or does he stroke her or engage in sexually provocative gestures towards her as he presents her – condescendingly, mockingly, and even vulgarly – as 'a quaint piece of beauty', with 'quaint' punning on 'the external female genitals' (3.5.53)?[68] Could an obscene gesture emphasize the sexual pun on 'doing', in Vindice's assertion to Gloriana that she should not worry about the 'disgrace' of an illicit rendezvous when ''Tis the best grace you have to do it well' (47)? Could a chilling caress accompany his blazon of the skull's features, including 'A pretty hanging lip, that has forgot how to dissemble' (56)? While such questions can only remain speculative, taking gestural liberties with the 'bony lady' would certainly not be a far stretch from dressing up Gloriana's bones, parading her as a 'concubine' (42), and holding mock conversation with her that is laced with contempt for women.

Indeed, Vindice's bitter reflections on his bony puppet soon conflate Gloriana with women in general in his expression of contumely for the entire sex. Vindice asks the skull, 'Does the silkworm expend her yellow labours / For thee? For thee does she undo herself'? (71–2); 'Does every proud and self-affecting dame / Camphor her face for this'? (83–4); do men turn thieves 'To refine such a thing'? (75–7). Likely pointing at or holding out the skull to the audience, he concludes, 'Here might a scornful and ambitious woman / Look through and

---

[66] Stallybrass, 'Reading the Body', 138–9, and Mullaney, 'Mourning and Misogyny', 259, among others, discuss the phallic connotations of the tongue, here. Stallybrass finds in this deathly kiss an 'inversion of sexual and social hierarchy' in that 'the trope of the female seducer, impersonated by a tongueless skull, inseminates the Duke with poison', and so 'the silent mouth of woman transfixes the tongue of masculine authority'. This inversion, however, does not gloss over the reality that Gloriana's remains are forced into the kind of sexual encounter she died avoiding. The Duchess draws attention to a connection between the Duke's tongue and genitals early in the play: 'Oh what it is to have an old-cool duke / To be as slack in tongue as in performance' (1.2.74–5).

[67] Thomas Middleton and William Rowley, *The Changeling*, ed. Gary Taylor and John Lavagnino, 1.1.237–8.

[68] *OED*, 'quaint, n.', 1.

through herself' (95–6). Vindice utterly degrades Gloriana's bones as the most harrowing and ugly vision of the nothingness all living material must become. Even worse, in making her skeleton his ultimate proof that all 'ladies' with their 'false forms / … deceive men but cannot deceive worms' (96–7), his illustration of women's foolish presumption in wearing rich attire, Vindice constructs an image of Gloriana entirely different from the woman whose 'purer part' refused to submit to the material temptations of a duke.

This severance of Gloriana's remains from any memory or association with 'her purer part' is very much wrapped up in Vindice's delight in demonstrating his own wit. Incessantly and emphatically in the passages cited above, Vindice directs our attention to the 'bare bone' of Gloriana ('for thee', 'for thee', 'for this', 'a thing', 'here', 'look', 'see' [84–96]). Vindice's rhetoric here depends entirely on the shocking spectacle of the skull that he has just unmasked to maximum dramatic effect, leaving a surprised Hippolito – who clearly expected to see a living woman under the '*tires*' and behind the mask – at a loss for words: 'Why brother, brother', is the only verbal response Hippolito can manage (49). Overall, Vindice celebrates his own wit and ingenuity. Wit and ingenuity are qualities of the mind, and the mind was often interchangeable with the soul or else considered the highest faculty of the soul.[69] Vindice uses Gloriana's skull as his wit's main prop rather than as a token of continued emotional or spiritual connection with her. He is giddily 'lost' in 'a throng of happy apprehensions' at the mere thought of how well 'suited' (both literally and figuratively) Gloriana is for the Duke in his revenge plot, and relishes sarcastically describing to Hippolito her 'delicious lip' and 'sparkling eye' (28–34). In a mock conversation with Gloriana, Vindice insinuates that Gloriana is seeking assurance that her affair will be 'secret', and he contemptuously answers, ''Twill be worth / Three velvet gowns to your ladyship' and 'Known? / Few Ladies respect that' (43–8). This pretend exchange strongly evokes a puppet master interpreting his puppet to the audience, and serves little purpose besides Vindice's enjoyment in performing and setting up the surprise of Gloriana's unmasking for Hippolito, who responds by 'applaud[ing]' the 'quaintness[70] of [his] malice, above thought' (107–8). Vindice takes equal delight in dramatically unmasking Gloriana to the agonizing Duke and in underlining the poetic justice of his death. Just as Antonio's unveiling of his wife before '*certain lords*' ensures that increased honour accrues to *his* name, both unmaskings of Gloriana are moments of triumph for Vindice, emphasizing his cunning rather than mournfully evoking the memory of the murdered Gloriana. Her skull and bones are emptied of spiritual significance in connection with Gloriana in order to serve Vindice's spirited wit.

---

[69]   For discussions of the immortality of the mind and of the mind and soul as interchangeable concepts in Plato (whose divisions of the soul were so influential to early modern thinkers), Aristotle, Augustine, and Aquinas, see Osmond, *Mutual Accusation*, 5–7, 16, and John P. Wright and Paul Potter (eds), *Psyche and Soma*, 46, 136–7, 142–3.

[70]   Brian Gibbons (ed.), *The Revenger's Tragedy*, glosses 'quaintness' here as 'witty ingenuity'.

While we cannot accurately describe an early modern audience's reactions to Vindice's treatment of the dead body of a loved one, if Hippolito's initial speechlessness at the sight of Gloriana dressed up is any indication, Vindice's unfeeling puppetry of the 'bony lady' held potential to disturb or create a feeling of uneasiness for the audience. Similar dramatic moments in other plays feature adverse responses much like Hippolito's in *The Revenger's Tragedy*. In *The Duke of Milan*, for example, when Francisco paints the cheeks, lips, and hands of Marcelia's corpse preparatory to deceiving the Duke, he pauses to ask his sister (whom he claims to be avenging in this act), 'How do you like my workmanship?' Far from approving, she responds, 'I tremble; / And thus to tyrannise upon the dead / Is most inhuman' (5.2.197–9). Similarly, in *The Lady's Tragedy*, when Govianus paints the dead Lady's face to poison the Tyrant, Govianus confides to the audience, 'A religious trembling shakes me by the hand / And bids me put by such unhallowed business' though 'revenge calls for't' (5.2.91–3). The soldiers' jokes evince their extreme discomfort with obeying the Tyrant's orders to disturb the Lady's body from its grave in the first place. One soldier fears that the corpse will 'rise / At the first jog' (4.3.76–7). The consequently 'abused' 'soul' of the Lady herself oversees the rescue of her corpse from the Tyrant's clutches (5.2.95), and onstage, her corpse and her ghost appear in identical attire. The ghost's concern for and visual connection to the corpse suggest a continuing link between lifeless body and departing soul, and a sense of this link is what gives Govianus and the soldiers such unease.[71] Even Hamlet, who himself handles Yorrick's skull, is troubled by the grave-diggers' rough treatment of what they unearth in their digging: 'That skull had a tongue in it and could sing once. How the knave jowls it to the ground, as if 'twere Cain's jawbone, that did the first murder!' (5.1.75–7), and the inscription over Shakespeare's own grave cursing 'he that moves my bones' is well known.[72] Staging uneasiness about disturbing dead bodies plausibly encouraged or elicited a similar unease from audience members, preventing them from dismissing Gloriana as empty material as brazenly as Vindice does. Vindice has intentionally plucked Gloriana's body from the basic dignity of Christian burial that even criminals facing execution were anxious to secure for themselves, believing the body's proper repose to be essential to the soul's peace and immortality.[73] Does the atmosphere of discomfort stem, in part, from a latent fear of repercussions for purposely disturbing the grave?

To examine the possibility of such repercussions, I turn to how Gloriana's physical presence as puppet onstage might signify in performance. Vindice repeatedly exploits the shock value of Gloriana's skull-face, first with the surprise

---

[71] The Tyrant, the only one who is comfortable with puppeting the Lady's corpse, notably dismisses any lingering connection between body and soul, claiming 'The house is hers, the soul is but a tenant' (5.2.3).

[72] See lxxvii in the General Introduction to Bevington's *Complete Works of Shakespeare*.

[73] See, for instance, Gittings, *Death, Burial, and the Individual*, 60–61.

unmasking before Hippolito and then with the 'dreadful' unmasking before the
dying Duke, at which point Vindice orders Hippolito closer with the torch, so 'that
[the Duke's] affrighted eyeballs / May start into those hollows' (3.5.146–7) of the
skull's eye-sockets. But is the frightful effect of Gloriana's staring 'hollows' always
under Vindice's precise control, as in these two carefully calculated unmaskings?
There is strong potential, I would argue, for the grim, unchanging skeleton face
to subtly undermine Vindice's exuberant glee at how he has cleverly 'fashioned'
Gloriana to serve in his revenge plot. And what is the effect of Gloriana's sombre,
fixed grin as Vindice unleashes his tirade against the vanity and deceptiveness of
women, holding her up as the support of his misogynistic rhetoric, casting her as
prostitute, and deriding her? Ironically, Vindice's puppeting of Gloriana's lifeless
body, by creating the illusion that she is animate, calls attention to what an animate
Gloriana's perspective *would be* on Vindice's role for her.

As puppet in Vindice's revenge show, moreover, Gloriana inherits the
puppet's associations with mockery. There is something grotesquely comic in
the incongruity of the stark skull-face peering out from rich attire. As Vindice
unloads his contempt for women onto Gloriana's skull and celebrates his ingenuity
in suiting her up for the Duke, her perpetual, gruesome grin could very easily
produce the effect of seeming to silently mock Vindice himself. Such mockery is
in keeping with the daring vulgarity and rebelliousness that came to be expected
from a puppet. At the same time, the belief in the corpse's continued importance to
the soul recalls and overlaps with what I have called the puppet's 'spiritual side',
that is, its earlier role in representing divine figures and its consequent association
with idolatry (and idolatry's attendant dangers), to give an edge of eeriness to
the puppet skull's derisive grin. Although Gloriana is so blatantly, exaggeratedly
material, then, she is not unambiguously material as it is understood in opposition
to the spiritual. In this ambiguity she poses a challenge to Vindice's flippant use
of her physical remains and to his contempt for women based on scorn for the
material as inferior to the spiritual.

The material, the feminine, and Death itself align in the figure of Gloriana,
according to Vindice's role for her in his revenge script, and in puppeting Gloriana,
Vindice appears as attempting, and finally failing, to control all three. In an allusion
to the traditional dance of death or danse macabre – visually depicted in familiar
scenes of an animated skeleton intruding upon the daily activities of people from
all levels of society to seize the person whose time it is to die – Vindice essentially
sets up his own scene of Death coming for the Duke.[74] In the dance of death

---

[74] Hans Holbein the Younger's 1538 publication of woodcuts marks perhaps the most
famous depiction of the danse macabre. The popularity of this series of illustrations is evident
in the several editions and imitations that followed: see Gundersheimer's introduction to
The Dance of Death by Hans Holbein, ix–x. For more information on the danse macabre,
see Sophie Oosterwijk, 'Of Corpses, Constables, and Kings', 61–90, which provides a
fascinating overview of the roots, development, and spread of the danse macabre through
various media (such as 'murals, stained glass windows, illuminated manuscripts, early
printed books, and sculpture'); Léonard P. Kurtz, *The Dance of Death and the Macabre*

scene Vindice creates, though, Gloriana is both the allegorical representation of the abstract concept of Death and Vindice's puppet and murder weapon. Here, the text underlines the arrogance of Vindice's assumption of absolute control over Gloriana's body and its signification by overlapping it with his assumption of control over Death itself. The scene that Vindice constructs reduces the usual allegorical representation of Death as a mysterious, often mocking, and entirely independent power (along with the remains of Gloriana's body) to a mere prop in Vindice's artistic murder. Vindice usurps Death's role in orchestrating every detail of the Duke's final moments – down to ensuring that he cannot even 'wink' to avoid the sight of his wife's adultery with his own bastard son. To emphasize his position as author of the Duke's death, Vindice pauses for reflection on the poetic justice of several of those details, such as the Duke's tongue rotting out after having caused Vindice's father 'grief' that 'made him die speechless' (3.5.196, 170). To the audience, the skeletal figure familiarly representative of Death loses its association with the unexpected to serve an entirely predictable role according to the plot that Vindice has previously outlined. Vindice's reduction of the traditional, allegorical representation of Death to a tool he physically and artistically controls in the authorship of his own dance of death scene resonates with the way he empties Gloriana's bones of spiritual potency and the way he associates the concept of divine justice or retribution with hollow stage effects.[75]

The play does not, however, entirely uphold this view of the material as void of spiritual significance or immaterial potency. Antonio's wife's rapist, the depraved Younger Son, clearly shares Vindice's opinion that 'wives', or women in general, 'are but made to go to bed and feed' (1.2.131). When the judge asks the Younger Son 'what moved you to't [the rape]', he callously replies, 'Why flesh and blood my lord: / What should move men unto a woman else?' (47–9), as if the only imaginable reason a man would concern himself with a woman would be to satisfy a carnal urge. The Younger Son's misogynistic reduction of women to the physical, combined with his flagrant disrespect for the justice system during his trial, leads to an interesting warning (albeit from fellow-misogynist Lussurioso) to 'play not with thy death' (53). In a sense, playing with Death is precisely what Vindice is doing too, both in taking justice into his own hands and in desecrating a woman's bodily remains.[76] Literally, in playing with the skeletal figure he is playing with the most familiar allegorical representation of Death, turning Death the skeleton, along with

---

Spirit, which also provides a useful overview, including a small section on the dance of death in England that lists numerous places and forms in which it appears; and Christian Kiening, 'Le Double décomposé', 1157–90, which considers, in the skeleton, the interplay between the abstract and the concrete, the image of oneself in death and Death itself.

[75] For Tanya Pollard, *Drugs and Theatre*, 113, the 'hollowing out of the female body is mirrored in the hollowing out of the interior worlds of the play's other characters as well'.

[76] C.f. Govianus's aside to the audience upon witnessing the Tyrant's use of the Lady's corpse to decorate his court: 'O who dares play with destiny but he / That wears security so thick upon him, / The thought of death and hell cannot pierce through' (*Lady's Tragedy* 5.2.57–9).

his former fiancée, into his personal puppet to serve his own agenda. But in doing so, Vindice forms part of yet another danse macabre scene that appears clearly to the audience, but that he himself does not consider. Much like the scholar in one of Holbein's famous woodcuts, who is oblivious to the presence of Death behind his own death's head or 'study's ornament' (the skeleton is actually holding up the skull to the distracted scholar in the illustration [Figure 1]), Vindice cannot see in Gloriana a symbol or warning of his own death. And yet Vindice, more often than anyone else, appears onstage with the skull or skeleton in tow, creating a striking allusion to the dance of death tradition and its visual depictions. In this light, Gloriana's perpetual grin – which I have read as having the effect of mocking Vindice when he draws attention to her skull-face as the main support for his misogynistic rant – gains additional significance. With the skull co-opted into a role that Gloriana died to avoid, the grin becomes eerie in terms of the skull's potential connection to the spirit of Vindice's murdered fiancée. But it is doubly eerie in that it also resembles the derisive grin of Death the skeleton as this figure integrates itself into the activities of its often unprepared and oblivious victims, on the verge of seizing them in depictions of the dance of death. In other words, the immaterial force of death (material only in its effects) conflates with the uncanny power of the skull in connection with Vindice's dead betrothed (I refer here both to the belief about the body's continuing link and importance to its departed soul and to the illusion of perspective produced by the animation of Gloriana's remains).

In using Gloriana's body as his tool and discounting the possibility of the spiritual potency of her relics, Vindice overlooks, to his own demise, the danger in playing with her. Hearing Antonio express 'wonder' at the murder of his enemies, Vindice cannot resist exclaiming, 'We may be bold / To speak it now: 'twas somewhat wittily carried / Though we say it. 'Twas we two [Vindice and Hippolito] murdered him!' (5.3.94–100). Tellingly, the same arrogant delight in his own ingenuity that governs Vindice's attempt to puppet Gloriana's body (and to puppet Death itself) also leads to the boastful confession that brings about his own death. Death is no longer Vindice's puppet, but regains its quality of unexpectedness: Vindice is baffled at Antonio's fatal response to his confession, and arguably the audience is also stunned by how carelessly Vindice betrays himself after executing a flawless revenge without incurring even a hint of suspicion. At the same time, the earlier images of Vindice unwittingly performing a dance of death subtly anticipate this moment.[77] Another such anticipatory moment is Vindice's orchestration of

---

[77]   In light of Vindice's position in his own dance of death scenes, the connection of Vindice with 'time' becomes interesting. Describing Vindice (as Piato) to the Duke, Hippolito claims, 'This our age swims within him; and if Time / Had so much hair I should take him for Time, / He is so near kin to this present minute' (1.3.24–6). As he is about to murder the Duke, Vindice incants, 'now nine years vengeance crowd into a minute' (3.5.121). While these references to time emphasize Vindice's determination to seize the opportune moment for revenge or 'hold' 'Occasion' by 'the fore-top', as he puts it (11.98–9), time, of course, often accompanies Death in its iconographic representations, as the grim reaper's scythe, for instance, or as an hourglass like the one tucked away in many of Holbein's dance of death illustrations.

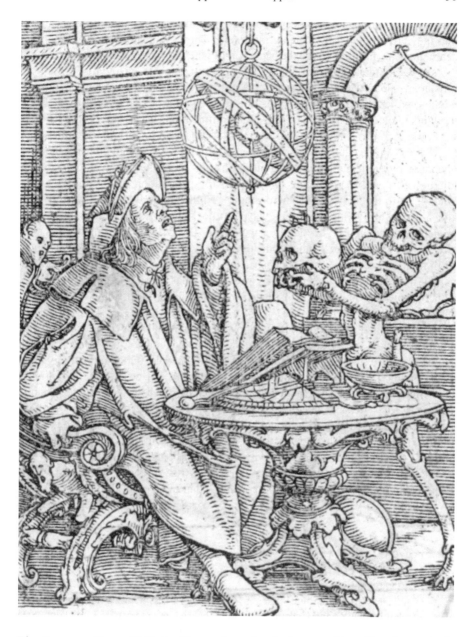

Fig. 1   From Holbein, Hans. *Les simulachres et historiées faces de la mort*. Lyon, 1538. This item is reproduced by permission of La Bibliothèque Nationale de France.

Lussurioso's and his nobles' deaths through yet another, literal dance of death in that they are murdered by dancing masquers. These moments keep the dance of death theme from slipping into the background with Gloriana's disappearance from the stage. Significantly, with Vindice's condemnation his misogynistic rhetoric falls apart, along with his control in dealing out death. Vindice's construction of women as 'leaky vessels'[78] in opposition to men who are 'made close' to 'keep thoughts in best' is evident in his oft-cited comment to Lussurioso, 'Tell but some woman a secret over night, / Your doctor may find it in the urinal i'the morning' (1.3.83–6). Vindice forces Gloriana's skull to represent women's treacherous openness by subjecting its poisonous mouth to the penetration of the Duke's tongue and possibly subjecting the skull to the penetration of his fingers as he holds it up to the audience's view onstage.[79] Mullaney finds that in 'master[ing]' and 'possess[ing]' Gloriana in this way, Vindice 'proves himself all male, not at all dependent upon or in the hands of women'.[80] But, as Mullaney also points out, after his perfect revenge Vindice is the one who 'cannot keep his mouth shut', thus spilling 'his secret, his carefully constructed maleness, and his life'.[81] Vindice, the puppet master, is finally overcome by precisely what he tried to puppet: both the construction of femaleness as distinct from and inferior to his male intelligence, and Death itself.

Overall, Vindice does not control or possess what remains of Gloriana's body as entirely as critics have previously asserted. Others have noted in Gloriana's silent stage presence a strange power or even a threat to Vindice, but do not perceive her as ever really escaping his control. Finin, for instance, discusses 'the potentially overwhelming presence of female power', which involves, through the very name 'Gloriana', the 'dread such a powerful female figure' as Queen Elizabeth 'evokes, threatening as she does to overwhelm masculine authority'. Finin focuses on Vindice's response to this power, his need and 'ability to manipulate Gloriana's remains with such mastery'.[82] Tanya Pollard brilliantly describes how 'in its very emptiness' the 'skull possesses a curious power', drawing attention to how 'Vindice implicitly likens' the skull's 'effect to that of alcohol'. Pollard explains:

---

[78] Paster, *Body Embarrassed*, Ch. 1.

[79] Mullaney, 'Mourning and Misogyny', 257, discusses 'Vindice's gross economy of tongue and genitalia', and Coddon, 'For show or useless property', 74–5, claims that Gloriana's 'mutilated state … evokes contemporary depictions of anatomized female corpses, and while her sexual organs have presumably long turned to dust, the fact that the skull kills with its "lips" suggests the *vagina dentate*, even without an actual vagina'. See also Stallybrass, 'Reading the Body', 139.

[80] Mullaney, 'Mourning and Misogyny', 259.

[81] Ibid.

[82] Finin, '"Wild Justice" and the Female Body', pars 1–3, 24.

Upon seeing her mouth, he claims, a drunkard would stop drinking, suggesting both that she would inspire a virtuous horror of death and, implicitly, that she would make drink unnecessary by replacing its effect.[83]

For Pollard, though, Vindice is immune to the intoxicating effect of Gloriana,[84] and his position as 'detached observer, contemptuously assessing the limited power of her morbid remains' serves as a 'model – albeit an imperfect one – for how to approach spectacles without either consuming or being consumed by their taint'.[85]

Conversely, I am arguing that Gloriana can be read as a warning against Vindice's detached and dismissive treatment of the material, a treatment clearly bound up in his subordinating view of women. Onstage, the material remains of Vindice's fiancée are not *empty* material. As Vindice animates Gloriana as his puppet and tool of revenge, the skull is also strangely animated by the puppet's associations with mockery and rebelliousness, seeming to escape Vindice's control and subvert his flood of misogynistic words through the blatant materiality he so contemptuously emphasizes. The puppet's grotesque derision and the danse macabre's chilling quality overlap in the skull's grin. And in Gloriana's case the puppet's associations with the spiritual – whether through its more distant liturgical role in representing the divine or through the spiritual dangers posed by the puppet as idol – merge with the superstition or belief about the departed soul's continued interest in the body. For some audience members, these associations held potential to be more than mere associations, and the dangers in using human remains unceremoniously as playthings – given added weight in that the skull was likely real and not a replica[86] – are in a sense confirmed by Vindice's death. Not only does Gloriana, as silent material, hold potential to mock Vindice, but, in his arrogant pleasure in manipulating and mastering her remains, Vindice is oblivious to having entered his own dance of death.

Gloriana is neither fully flesh nor fully spirit; as a human relic with a haunting effect on the audience, she occupies an intermediary position between the two. She is uncanny in the Jentschien sense of the uncanny resulting from uncertainty as to 'whether an apparently animate being is really alive' or 'whether a lifeless object might not be in fact animate'.[87] In this uncanniness, she poses a wordless threat or warning, unheeded by Vindice but not necessarily lost upon the audience. Other women represented onstage share this threatening uncanniness. Frances Dolan discusses the possibility of a darker and menacing side to Hermione's perhaps vindictive ghostliness in the final scene of *The Winter's Tale*.[88] Leontes's hesitation

---

[83]   Pollard, *Drugs and Theatre*, 117.

[84]   For insightful analyses of consumption and decay, poison and corrosiveness in the play, refer to Stallybrass, 'Reading the Body', and Pollard, *Drugs and Theatre*.

[85]   Pollard, *Drugs and Theatre*, 117, 122.

[86]   See Rist, *Revenge Tragedy*, 10.

[87]   Sigmund Freud, 'The Uncanny', 421.

[88]   Frances Dolan, 'Hermione's Ghost', 227–9.

to touch Hermione[89] indeed suggests his fear at the moment the supposed statue steps off its pedestal, a moment which confuses categories of inanimate and animate and also matter and spirit: is the now moving figure a statue stirred by magic, Hermione's ghost, or something else? Susan Carter's corpse holds a similar uncanny power that quite unnerves her murderer in *The Witch of Edmonton*. After Susan's ghost appears on either side of her bigamous husband's bed, ghastly staring him in the face, her corpse is carried to his bedside – with one eye open, also staring him in the face. The audience might half-expect her corpse to sit up and accuse him, especially since the actor's body, now portraying a lifeless corpse, was only seconds ago standing upright as Susan's ghost. The already-spooked Frank cannot bear the sight of the body, pleading, 'For pity's sake, remove her'.[90] Interestingly, before murdering her, Frank attempted to make Susan a kind of puppet-wife, wedding her to keep up appearances of obedience to his father through a socially approved marriage, merely in order to secure finances for himself and his real wife, Winnifrede. Frank objectifies Susan as a mere instrument in his plot to deceive his father, and ends up murdering her out of sheer annoyance when, as he tries to take his leave of her, she will not stop talking, expressing her emotions as a new wife. Prior to her murder, Frank reveals that he considers Susan as nothing but his 'whore', since, unbeknownst to her, Frank already has a wife, which invalidates his marriage with Susan. Correspondingly, before Hermione's apparent death and uncanny reappearance in *The Winter's Tale*, Leontes calls her a 'thing' too vulgar to name. Although she interprets the tribulation she must endure as 'for my better grace', her spiritual constancy and integrity do not prevent Leontes from casting her away as a defiled object (2.1.83, 123). I discussed earlier how Vindice perceives Gloriana as 'body' both before and after her death. While the uncanny collapse of matter and spirit does not seem a particularly productive or useful source of power for women if it can only be effected through their skeletons, corpses, or a seeming return from the dead, arguably these instances of the uncanny are so unsettling because, in blurring the line between material and immaterial, they confuse the categories so instrumental in subordinating and dismissing women.

At a time when, with the progression of religious reform, sharper lines were being drawn between body and soul and between the material and the immaterial, the early modern stage remained a place where, with the necessarily physical representation of spirits or ghosts – or the use of a special fabric to signify a concept of the immaterial, such as 'a robe for to goo invisibell' – these lines were quite fluid.[91] As women were increasingly relegated to the inferior side of this deepening

---

[89]   William Shakespeare, *The Winter's Tale*, ed. David Bevington, 5.3.107–9. Paulina must prod Leontes, 'Nay, present your hand. / When she was young you wooed her. Now in age / Is she become the suitor?'

[90]   Thomas Dekker, John Ford, and William Rowley, *The Witch of Edmonton*, ed. Peter Corbin and Douglas Sedge, 4.2.149. Subsequent references to the play cite this edition.

[91]   For an investigation into what such a robe – which we know Philip Henslowe 'laid out part of a £3 10s sum' for – might look like or be made from, refer to Barbara Palmer, 'Staging Invisibility in English Early Modern Drama', 113–28.

body-soul divide and in a genre often noted for its pronounced misogyny, this capacity for and even tendency towards blurring distinctions between the physical and spiritual could open a space for questioning, undermining, and even warning against, as in the case of Gloriana, the dismissal of the physical as empty of and inferior to the spiritual.

Bartholomew Fair's Puppets and Ursula's 'Greasy Soul'

> To persuade any matter we intend, or to stirre up any passion in a multitude, if we can aptly confirme our opinion or intention with any visible object, no doubt but the persuasion would be more forcible, and the passion more potent.
> – Thomas Wright, *The Passions of the Minde* (5.1.156–7)

The puppet Dionysius, engaged in a heated and hilariously absurd debate with Zeal-of-the-land Busy over its own status as 'idol', notoriously silences Busy by lifting its garments to reveal its sexlessness beneath. Busy's 'main argument against' the puppet is that he is 'an abomination, for the male among you putteth on the apparel of the female, and the female of the male' (5.5.55, 82–4, sd between 90–91). The sexlessness Dionysius claims in answer to Busy is represented by 'the mere wood and cloth of the puppet's body, or perhaps the smooth flesh of the puppeteer's forearm'.[92] In the latter scenario, Puppet Dionysius is not just exposing its puppet-body; rather, according to the analogy that equates puppet and puppeteer, or tool and artist, with body and soul, the puppet is ultimately lifting its body to expose its inner animating force, revealing that force to be both physical and beyond gender. In *Bartholomew Fair*, as in *The Revenger's Tragedy*, the performance of puppetry works to collapse the hierarchy of gender as it discursively connects to the hierarchy of soul over body. This section of the chapter seeks to investigate the links between Dionysius's final moment of triumph and the play's representations of female characters.

In his seminal article on '*Bartholomew Fair* and Its Puppets', Jonas Barish reads the play as bringing everything, including and especially the soul, to the level of gross physicality. He analyzes a 'series of tropes which reduce first the brain and then the soul itself to the level of physicality'. These tropes include Wasp's vision of the interior of Cokes's head as 'hung with cockel-shells, pebbles, fine wheat-straws, and here and there a chicken's feather and a cobweb' (1.5.83–5); Quarlous's reference to 'a spoonful of brain' (123); and Wasp's exasperated wish that his own 'brains' had been 'bowled at, or threshed out' when he first decided to take on Cokes as his charge (3.4.40–42).[93] Most notably, Edgeworth 'degrades the soul itself to the level of matter' in scoffing at Cokes: 'Talk of him to have a soul? 'Heart, if he have any more than a thing given him instead of salt, only to

---

[92] Shershow, *Puppets*, 104.
[93] Barish, '*Bartholomew Fair* and Its Puppets', 4.

keep him from stinking, I'll be hanged afore my time presently' (4.2.46–8).[94] For Barish, 'with this view of the soul as a kind of preservative in the blood, placed there to keep the body from putrefaction, the reduction of the spirit to the flesh is complete'.[95] This emphasis on the 'reduction', 'degradation', or 'debasement' of the spirit to the level of the material has become a critical commonplace in interpretive engagement with *Bartholomew Fair*,[96] and understandably so, given Jonson's 'special decorum' in deliberately staging the play at the Hope. The Hope was also used for the cruel practice of bear-baiting, was 'as dirty as Smithfield' – where Bartholomew Fair was held – and 'as stinking every whit' (Induction 134–5). The coarseness of the language matches the filth of the physical playhouse – Puppet Leander's retort to Leatherhead the puppeteer, '*kiss my hole here and smell*', serves as a prime example (5.4.114–15). The articles the Scrivener adumbrates in the contract between Jonson and the audience include one holding that audience members who 'shall so desperately or ambitiously play the fool … to challenge the author of scurrility because the language somewhere savours of Smithfield, the booth, and the pig-broth' must forfeit themselves to ridicule (Induction 125–8). The notion of language having a distinct taste seems to physicalize the abstraction of language itself.[97]

But, at the same time, the insistent critical emphasis on the play's reduction or degradation of the soul to the level of flesh (and for Jonson, language was also very much connected to the soul[98]) assumes and maintains the hierarchy of spirit over matter. In this way, critics have overlooked how *Bartholomew Fair* actually works to undo this divide in its defence of the theatre. Indeed, the frequent vulgarity and emptiness of language throughout the play argues for an imperfection or impurity of soul or spirit that everywhere accompanies displays of the physically gross or base. Thomas Cartelli's reading of the fair as a 'gray world' is suggestive here:

---

[94]   Ibid.

[95]   Ibid.

[96]   See also, for instance, the same argument in Mathew R. Martin, *Between Theater and Philosophy*, 134: the play's 'pungent physicality', he states, 'bringing the high low and reducing the spiritual to the material, equates authority and judgment … with folly and flatulence. The play appropriates the strategies of what Bakhtin labels "grotesque realism," whose essential principle is "degradation; that is, the lowering of all that is high, spiritual, abstract; it is the transfer to the material level, to the sphere of earth and the body"'.

[97]   This idea of language having a 'savour', of course, is not unusual in Jonson, who delights elsewhere in the metaphor of language or writing as a feast that he, as the author/cook, has served up for his audience (see, for instance, the Prologue to *The New Inn*, or the Epistle in the front matter of *Volpone*).

[98]   In *Timber or Discoveries*, ed. Ralph S. Walker, 45–6, for instance, Jonson writes that 'Language most shows a man: "speak that I may see thee". It springs out of the most retired and inmost parts of us, and is the image of the parent of it, the mind'. In the preface to the masque *Hymenaei*, ed. Stephen Orgel, he describes the 'riches and magnificence in the outward celebration or show' of a masque as its body, and the poetry, or 'high and hearty inventions to furnish the inward parts', as its soul.

Whereas Shakespeare takes his characters on a kind of therapeutic vacation halfway out of this world in order to make them whole, Jonson rubs the faces of his characters in the dirt of this-worldly experience in order to relieve them of their pretensions and unnaturalness, to make them, if not whole, at least a bit more acclimated to 'things as they are'.[99]

Instead of having a debasing influence, coming to terms with the physical might exercise a corrective or restorative effect on spiritual haughtiness and hypocrisy.[100] Certainly the idea that the body corrupts and drags down the soul was the dominant view, but in emphasizing this convention we tend to oversimplify, forgetting the early modern understanding of the soul as itself deeply flawed. The idea that the stain of original sin inheres in all souls (except for Christ's and the virgin Mary's) is entrenched in Christian doctrine, Protestant and Catholic, and the poetic genre of the body-soul dialogue imagines the soul and body engaged in an unresolvable dispute about which one is ultimately responsible for leading the whole person towards damnation. In a text Jonson was certainly familiar with, *The Passions of the Minde in Generall*, Thomas Wright devotes book 6 to 'the defects or imperfections of mens soules'.[101] He discusses the 'blindnesse' and limitations of the mind as proof of the soul's imperfection, and after elaborating upon various forms of error and ignorance to which the mind is prone, Wright notes that while some gaps in knowledge might be excusable, such as, for instance, ignorance about divine matters, people 'at least' might have 'knowne themselves; for what was more neere them then their owne soules and bodies ... ? Yet the Ignorance and Errours, which ... inveigle us, are almost incredible'.[102] For Wright, failure to truly know oneself (a weakness that plagues almost everyone in *Bartholomew Fair*) signals the flawed nature of the soul.

Bartholomew Fair does not appeal to any initial concept of the soul as superior to the flesh in order to stage a process of debasement. Instead, it presents various images and examples of the immaterial as insubstantial and void of meaning. John Littlewit, for example, shares with Vindice a delight in pointing out and celebrating his own wit and artistic creativity – qualities attributed to the soul – but as his name signals and his shallow and pointless puns confirm, little is worth celebrating. We first meet Littlewit applauding himself for 'A pretty conceit, and worth the finding!' (1.1.1). This 'conceit' is the coincidence that Bartholomew Cokes has taken forth

---

[99]   Thomas Cartelli, '*Bartholomew Fair* as Urban Arcadia', 157.

[100]   Leah S. Marcus, *Politics of Mirth*, 57–8, offers a related assessment of the fair's paradoxically curative effect: 'Smithfield swirls with madness and disorder, but it is a madness that cures the mad. By bringing lost souls back to reason, the fair in fact recapitulates a specialty of its namesake St. Bartholomew, who was noted above all as a healer of the mad'.

[101]   Jonson, who may have met Wright in 1598 while in prison, wrote a commendatory poem for the 1604 edition of *Passions*. See David W. Kay, *Ben Jonson: A Literary Life*, 28–9.

[102]   Wright, *Passions of the Minde*, 297, 300.

a marriage licence to marry Grace Wellborn on Bartholomew Day. The 'device' of 'Bartholomew upon Bartholomew', as Littlewit puts it, is enough to elate him at the 'luck' he has 'to spin out these fine things still and like a silk-worm, out of myself' (1–2, 6–7). The proctor's opinion of his own wit gives him a marked superiority complex: 'Who would have marked such a leap-frog chance now?' he asks, as though he is the only one to perceive the obvious coincidence, and he is always explicitly drawing attention to his little quibbles with self-congratulatory remarks: 'there now, I speak quib too', 'There I am again, la!', 'Good!', and 'There I am again!' all appear in his first speech alone (7–8, 13–15, 25, 27). Littlewit is an author-figure as writer of the puppet play, but the 'inspiration' he provides to animate the puppet players is hardly superior to their materiality (5.5.94). In fact, his script is drowned out when Leatherhead, the puppeteer, lets Dionysius's pure materiality answer Busy's charges (and this materiality proves to be the most effective answer).

Littlewit's authorship of the puppet play and his conviction of his superior wit correspond with his arrogant presumption in puppeting his wife. He dresses up his 'little pretty Win' like his doll to show off to others (5.6.12), as when he shows her to Winwife in a 'habit' she 'would not ha' worn' on her own, asking 'Does't not fine, Master Winwife?' (1.2.3–5). As if Win were his object to share, Littlewit also orders her to kiss his friends despite her obvious discomfort. 'I envy no man my delicates, sir' (11), he explains to Winwife upon instructing Win to let Winwife kiss her. When Win protests at Quarlous's unsolicited kiss, asking her husband to 'help' her, to her dismay ('you are a fool, John') Littlewit insists she comply with 'our worshipful good friends' and kiss Quarlous again (1.3.32–43). Needing an excuse to attend the fair despite the Puritan disapproval of his mother-in-law, Dame Purecraft, and her suitor, Busy, Littlewit has Win feign a craving for roast pig. When Win becomes inconvenient for him at the fair, he simply deposits her in Ursula's tent for safekeeping. To Littlewit, Win is a pretty doll he can pass around, brag about, use as a decoy, and then set down somewhere when he is finished with her to take up again at his later convenience.

The game of 'vapours', so enjoyed by Wasp and Knockem, together with Busy's obsession with the 'spirit', join Littlewit's shallow wit as further examples of the immaterial as disappointingly empty. Knockem's favourite word, 'vapours', occurs 69 times in *Bartholomew Fair*.[103] While in one sense, 'vapours' is a word for 'a fancy or fantastic idea; a foolish brag or boast', the word also resonates with humoural theory, as Patrick Grant suggests.[104] Lemnius, in *The Touchstone*

---

[103] Patrick Grant, *Literature and the Discovery of Method*, 72.

[104] *OED*, 4. The *OED* cites *Bartholomew Fair* as an example of this meaning. *OED*, 3. *pl.* a, also defines 'vapours' as 'In older medical use: Exhalations supposed to be developed within the organs of the body (esp. the stomach) and to have an injurious effect upon the health'. Examples include a 1530 reference to 'humours and vapours that styre and move the ... phantasye' and a 1639 reference to 'ill vapours of the stomach' that cause the 'head' to 'ache'.

of Complexions (1576), explains 'the Spirite is a certayne vapour, effluence or expyration, proceding out of the humours',[105] and in 1615 Helkiah Crooke defines spirit as 'a subtle and thin body always movable, engendered of blood and vapour, and the vehicle or carriage of the faculties of the soul'.[106] Significantly, 'vapours', in their connection with 'spirit' – understood not as an alternative word for 'soul' but as a 'corporeall' vehicle of 'the finest and subtillest susbstance', a vehicle the soul uses to 'execute her offices'[107] – occupy an intermediary position between the physical and the immaterial. Although in humoural context the term 'vapours' refers to an ethereal force connected to the soul, in the play vapours ultimately amount to a combination of tobacco fumes with the heady influence of '*nonsense*' (4.4.24–5 sd). The actual '*game of vapours*' that takes place in act 4 calls for '*every man to oppose the last man that spoke, whether it concerned him or no*' (sd). The cantankerous Wasp seems to be playing a perpetual game of vapours with everyone he encounters, while Knockem inserts the word 'vapours' into his every utterance until the word becomes completely meaningless. And yet, the absurdity or 'travesty of reason' that 'vapours' represent is a weakness that cannot be attributed solely to the '*physical* excess' of 'humours, ale, and tobacco'.[108] Instead, in their humoural sense, vapours participate in a mysterious mingling of elements of body and soul. Elusive in both meaning and substance, 'vapours' provide a contrast to the fair's juicy physicality, but not the moral contrast of pure spirit with sullied flesh. The play's sustained comic attention to vapours thus problematizes the view that *Bartholomew Fair* presents the soul's degradation to the level of the physical.

Busy's very different invocations of the 'spirit' are just as void of meaning as Knockem's constant references to 'vapours'. Busy claims:

> I was moved in spirit to be here this day in this Fair, this wicked and foul Fair, and fitter may it be called a foul than a Fair. To protest against the abuses of it, the foul abuses of it, in regard of the afflicted saints that are troubled, very much troubled, exceedingly troubled, with the opening of the merchandise of Babylon again, and the peeping of popery upon the stalls here, here, in the high places. See you not Goldilocks, the purple strumpet there? In her yellow gown and green sleeves? The profane pipes, the tinkling timbrels? A shop of relics! (3.6.75–83)

Jonson is poking fun, here, at the hyperbole and repetition of public preaching, but Busy's 'spirit'-inspired ramblings also betray an enjoyment of his own speech not unlike Littlewit's pleasure at his own 'conceits'. He holds onto certain words as if he particularly likes their effect ('fair', 'foul', 'trouble' – and 'exceedingly' in almost

---

[105]   Qtd in Grant, *Literature and the Discovery of Method*, 68.

[106]   Crooke, *Mikrokosmographia*, book 3, Ch. 12, 173. Crooke breaks down and explains this definition in complex detail on 174–5.

[107]   Ibid., book 3, Ch. 12, 174; book 1, Ch. 4, 10.

[108]   Martin, *Between Theater and Philosophy*, 135, emphasis added.

every speech), giving the impression that he awkwardly makes up his objections as he speaks. Busy also decorates with alliteration wherever possible and often strews his rants with loose biblical allusions of a high-sounding, condemnatory strain but stale in his anti-Catholic invective, as with his construction of Trash with her gingerbread as the whore of Babylon, here, with her 'merchandise' of 'popery'. In short, Busy's rants of the 'spirit', or 'sanctified noise', as he puts it, are as crowded with empty rhetoric and superficial decoration as Wasp imagines Cokes's head to be crowded with feathers and cockleshells and other vain trifles.[109]

Busy's exaggerated hypocrisy ultimately exposes the privileging of the 'spirit' over the body as a false pretence in service of self-righteousness and, in particular, of masculine self-righteousness. Entering into 'disputation' with Puppet Dionysius after interrupting the puppet show, Busy again announces, 'I will not fear to make my spirit and gifts known! Assist me, zeal, fill me, fill me; that is, make me full' (5.5.26, 35–6). Questioned by the puppet as to whether his '*calling*' is '*lawful*', he answers, 'Yes, mine is of the spirit' (46–8). Of course, Busy is obviously only 'moved in spirit' to 'make' himself 'full' of Ursula's roast pig. Just before Busy enters the stage for the first time, Littlewit informs us that he 'found [Busy] fast by the teeth i' the cold turkey-pie' (1.6.31). Even after this snack, as soon as the prospect of eating Bartholomew pig presents itself, Busy fixates on the pig as something that 'may be eaten, very exceeding well eaten' (46). He comes up with a ridiculous justification for 'the public eating of swine's flesh' – it will 'profess our hate and loathing of Judaism' – enabling him to conclude, 'I will therefore eat, yea, I will eat exceedingly' (83–5). Busy then centres on pig as the 'only' item 'not comprehended in my admonition' of the fair (3.6.25), and correspondingly on the 'good titillation of the famelic sense, which is the smell' (the stage direction indicates that '*Busy scents after* [the pig] *like a hound*') – a sense which Busy claims it is 'a sin of obstinacy' to 'decline or resist' (3.2.70–72). Of course, all the remaining senses must be blocked from the idolatry of the fair at all costs (Busy orders his group to 'Look not toward' Leatherhead's 'wares of devils' and to 'harken not' to his advertising cries [3.2.34–6]). When they have finally left Ursula's booth, Busy, who ate 'two and a half' pigs, has not shaken the craving:

> PURECRAFT: Brother Zeal-of-the-land! What shall we do? My Daughter, Win-the-fight, is fallen into her fit of longing again.
>
> BUSY: For more pig? There is no more, is there? (3.6.43, 34–6)

Despite his over-the-top hypocrisy, Busy is in a sense correct in attributing his presence at the fair to the 'spirit', in that appetite or desire was often attributed

---

[109] Marcus, *Politics of Mirth*, 38–63, demonstrates that Busy's hypocrisy stems from 'deficient self-knowledge' as part of a larger discussion about how the play critiques various abuses of authority (in an ambivalent but eloquent defence of James's authority) and forwards a message of recognizing one's own faults before condemning others.

to the soul.[110] Indeed, in the genre of body-soul dialogue, a familiar complaint of the body to its soul is that the soul is responsible for first corrupting its once innocent flesh by bringing to it unwholesome desire. But Busy is busy covering up his own urges by projecting them onto the female body, and more specifically, onto Win. The 'disease of longing', he preaches, 'is a disease, a carnal disease, or appetite, incident to women', and as he is about to enter Ursula's tent, Busy announces to Littlewit, 'Enter the tents of the unclean for once, and satisfy your wife's frailty. Let your frail wife be satisfied' (1.6.42–3, 3.2.74–5). Littlewit's plan for getting to the fair relies on the common assumption that women, especially pregnant women, are extra-susceptible to the weaknesses and desires of the body. Pregnant women's susceptibility to cravings was perhaps too ingrained a cultural assumption to be subverted, here, but Win does not really crave anything at the fair. In order to satisfy their own cravings, a blatant hypocrite (Busy) and a shallow wit (Littlewit) are the ones who construct Win as particularly subject to the frailties of the flesh due to her gender and suggested pregnancy. At the very least, this plot detail demonstrates awareness of the hypocrisy and shallowness built into the stereotype.

At first, this subtle critique of the assumption that women were more prone than men to the influence of the body seems insignificant alongside the sheer presence of Ursula. Hailed as the 'Body o' the Fair' and 'fatness of the Fair', Ursula specializes in satisfying cravings for flesh, providing, for a price, both pigs to eat and women to have sex with (2.5.65, 2.2.106, 2.5.36–7). The excessively corpulent 'pig-woman' and 'she-bear'[111] of the fair is herself a manifestation of the fluidity in her tent between human flesh for sexual consumption and animal flesh to eat. After scalding herself with drippings from her roasting pan during her furious attack on Quarlous and Winwife, she even calls for 'some cream and salad oil' to treat her wound (2.5.145). This request, as Alexander Leggatt observes, gives the impression that she herself is an oversized slab of food that has just

---

[110] Appetite or desire could be considered a subdivision of the will (usually accepted as a faculty of the soul) or a separate and lower faculty of the soul in itself that was more closely aligned with the body and could strive against the will. Osmond, *Mutual Accusation*, 5–6, finds that conflicting positions in separate works of Plato as to whether 'the appetitive faculty is part of the soul, and hence desires logically come from it', or desires are 'a phenomena of the body that can struggle against the soul', are a main source of the 'uncertainty' providing 'the intellectual essence of the body and soul debates. Who tempts? Who executes?' See also 14–16, 37, and Wright and Potter, *Psyche and Soma*, 46.

[111] 2.2.64, 2.3.1. Ursula's name, of course, as modern editors point out, associates her both with the bear star Ursa Major and (as the largest figure on the stage) with the bears that were cruelly baited in the same theatre in which the play was performed. Helen Ostovich, in the headnote for 2.5, points out that Ursula is also connected with pigs through her association with 'Demeter of the Thesmophoria, or Eleusinian Mysteries: the Sow-goddess, goddess of women. Her worshippers, like the Thesmophoriazusae in Aristophanes's play, celebrated the return of Persephone from Hades by purifying and sacrificing pigs, roasting and devouring them as a kind of sacrament'.

been cooked and is about to be seasoned.[112] Something about Ursula's undeniably extreme fleshliness, however, strangely undoes the conventional opposition between spirit and flesh, an undoing that culminates with Puppet Dionysius's victory in his 'disputation' with Busy.

In contravention to the familiar trope of the body as a restrictive cage for the soul, Ursula's body and everything around her is uncontained. She is so unmanageably large that she must have her chair 'let out o' the sides ... that [her] hips might play' (2.2.58–9); her vulgar language, 'greasier than her pigs', flows from her as endlessly as her shiny sweat (2.5.116);[113] she feels as if she will 'melt away to the first woman, a rib' (2.2.47–8); Knockem, too, jokes that 'vexing' Ursula in 'this hot weather' will amount to 'melting down a pillar of the Fair' (2.3.45–7); and her pigs roast until they sweat, their eyes pop out, and they are about to fall from the spit. As if exercising a strange, intangible influence, Ursula powerfully entices people to her tent from far and wide with nothing more substantial than a scent on the wind. Every character ends up in Ursula's tent at one point, either lured there or compelled by bodily need, as with Mistresses Littlewit and Overdo, who must enter her tent to relieve themselves. Something ubiquitous and inescapable thus emanates from Ursula and her tent and the corporeality, both succulent and disgusting, that she represents. Ursula's immaterial power of enchantment, furthermore, and her ability to provide assistance to women (albeit in a very rough and short-lived manner, considering she ends up trying to enlist them as prostitutes) are part of what links her to sorceress and goddess figures. Her status as pig-woman luring customers to her booth to become drunk and over-indulge their carnal appetites connects her to the enchantress Circe, who turned men into swine,[114] while her constant cooking fire at the centre of the fair community, which causes her to sweat profusely and 'water the ground in knots as I go like a great garden pot' (2.2.48–9), links her to hearth-goddess and fertility-goddess figures.[115] Ursula even resembles a fury brandishing a flaming torch or scourge when she emerges from her fire with the scalding pan to chase away Quarlous and Winwife (Winwife even ridicules her before the attack as 'Mother o' the Furies, I think, by her fire-brand' [2.5.67]). These overlapping allusions paradoxically infuse the fleshly Ursula with an incorporeal potency that has nothing to do with moral purity.

Instead, impurity reigns at the fair. Jonathan Haynes draws our attention to a 'theme of adulteration' in the play:[116] Ursula adulterates tobacco with 'coltsfoot'

---

[112]   Alexander Leggatt, *English Renaissance Comedy*, 140.

[113]   Critics have commented on the vulgarity of Ursula's language matching the grossness of her physical appearance. See, for example, Mary W. Bledsoe, 'The Function of Linguistic Enormity', 153.

[114]   Refer to Melinda Gough, 'Jonson's Siren Stage', for a full discussion of Jonson's treatment of Circean and siren myth in his defence of the theatre from Puritan anti-theatricalists.

[115]   Neil Rhodes, *Elizabethan Grotesque*, 146, links Ursula to Demeter, in particular.

[116]   Jonathan Haynes, *Social Relations of Jonson's Theater*, 123.

and mixes ale with extra froth (2.2.84), while Trash supposedly blends 'stale bread, rotten eggs, musty ginger, and dead honey' into her gingerbread (2.2.8–9). This adulteration aligns thematically with the play's insistence on the mutual adulteration of body and soul, as opposed to the critically favoured idea of the staged degradation of the soul. As already mentioned, in body-soul dialogues the body often holds the soul responsible for corrupting it with desire. In this light, Ursula's description of herself as 'all fire and fat' is significant. Flame and light are, of course, traditional symbols for the soul.[117] While Ursula's fat melts away before the fire, the fire is fed by such fat and oil, suggesting the fatal inextricability of body and soul. Ursula certainly does not view herself as flesh alone: 'I can but hold life and soul together with this [ale] ... and a whiff of tobacco, at most' (2.2.74–5), she tells Nightingale, here again underlining the fusion of the body and soul in her notion that her physical vices are what feed her soul and keep it from departing.

Jonson's constant and creative emphasis on Ursula's 'fatness' in her every mention and appearance relishes the flesh in all its excesses. Gail Kern Paster, however, has pointed out that Bakhtinian readings of Ursula and her booth's bodiliness as 'part of the play's apparent celebration of Carnival' problematically overlook 'cultural norms that distinguish sharply between the bodily "needs" of men and women'.[118] 'Only female characters', for instance, need to undergo the humiliation of asking for a chamber-pot, because 'unlike [*The Winter's Tale*'s] Autolycus or any other male character in this period who needs to urinate, they cannot merely "look upon" the nearest stage property hedge but are tied by the invisible leading strings of culture to a concealed receptacle'.[119] Ursula's chamber-pot thus makes her 'the instrument of patriarchy', according to Paster, in that once Win and Mistress Overdo are constrained by cultural norms to 'seek out the booth as privy', the booth, as 'central locus of desire in the fair', continues to serve 'prevailing cultural requirements in transforming the women from subjects

---

[117] Flame as symbolic of the soul is perhaps most evident in familiar descriptions of death as a 'snuffing' out, as when Othello famously extinguishes a torch, lantern, or candle before killing Desdemona, reflecting, as he does so, that he will 'Put out the light, and then put out the light' of Desdemona's soul. The flame as metaphor for the soul, a spark of divinity animating human clay, is of course also familiar from Promethean myth, as Othello himself points out: 'Should I repent me; but once put out thy light, / ... / I know not where is that Promethean heat / That can thy light relume' (5.2.7–13). Francis Quarles's *Hieroglyphikes of the Life of Man* and Robert Farlie's *Lychnocausia*, both books of emblems, are entirely devoted to images of a candle and flame (or snuffed-out flame and smoke), which refer explicitly to the body-soul relationship, likening body to tallow and soul to flame. Ursula is referred to as both 'tallow' and 'oil' and as an oily 'lamp' (2.5.69, 114, 2.2.106–7). She shares this quality with Falstaff, who, after Gadshill, 'sweats to death, / And lards the lean earth as he walks along' (*1 King Henry IV* 2.2.107–8).

[118] Paster, *Body Embarrassed*, 36.

[119] Ibid.

to objects', as Ursula tries to enlist them as prostitutes.[120] Ursula also supports and perpetuates patriarchal culture when, in response to the taunts of Quarlous and Winwife, most of the insults she can think of are decidedly misogynistic. She claims, for example, the men are 'poxed' from 'lean playhouse poultry that has the bony rump sticking out like the ace of spades' (2.5.91–2). Although Ursula's body itself is uncontained, her habits of thought are constrained by the cultural construction of the female body as a site of shame.

And yet Ursula's body also lends a spirit of mirth to her language. This mirth does not make Ursula a wholesome character – she has no qualms, for instance, about cheating her customers with adulterated tobacco and ale to make more money, or about raising the price of her ware if the customer happens to be 'a great-bellied wife' who 'long[s] for't' (2.2.100–101). But with her friends and before the audience, Ursula repeatedly and comically draws attention to her size. She comments on her intolerance for the heat of her profession, imagining herself as a giant gardening can watering the ground with sweat, or claiming she will soon melt down to a rib; expresses exasperation at squeezing into a chair too small for her hips; compares her bulk to her servant's 'grasshopper's thighs' (61); and so on. Her flesh itself represents a certain immaterial generosity in that, in a Falstaffian vein, she offers it as a source of laughter, the butt of her own jokes. This generosity contrasts sharply with Quarlous and Winwife, who, like vicious dogs baiting the 'she-bear' for entertainment, cruelly provoke her to the point of physical injury by jeering at her obesity. Ursula is herself fully 'adulterated': she good-naturedly pokes fun at her own body, but becomes violent when strangers joke about it, and disparages the female body in general in her impatience and anger. She exploits other women and yet shows a glimmer of compassion in begrudgingly providing her chamber-pot. She is excessively corpulent, but she is also the wielder of the light, warmth, and flame at the heart of the fair, the spark and fire that animates many other characters, drawing them inside her tent, where they show their true colours in their interactions with one another. Overall, Ursula's abundant corpulence cannot be read as unequivocally conveying a negative view of the flesh.

As the play's most extreme example of the cultural association between women and flesh, Ursula demonstrates a certain spiritedness, suggesting that the flesh should not always be considered in opposition to the soul and that the soul can be present without being superior to and purer than the flesh, and thus degraded by it. Jonson, whose conversion to Catholicism in 1598 may have lasted 12 years,[121] is even more explicitly playing with and poking fun at conflicting notions of the body-soul relationship through Zeal-of-the-land Busy (who is constantly spewing empty anti-Catholic rhetoric) and Bartholomew Cokes (who represents a kind of naïve, uncritical version of Catholic thinking) and what the puppets represent for

---

[120]   Ibid., 37.
[121]   Richard Harp, 'Catholicism', in 'Jonson and His Era', 112.

each of them.[122] G.M. Pinciss establishes Cokes's connection to Catholicism by persuasively arguing that, just as Banbury is an 'appropriate' area of residence for Busy, being 'a town in Oxfordshire closely identified in the public mind with both cakes and Puritan extremism', Cokes's frequently mentioned residence in Harrow on the Hill is not without meaning. 'The association of Harrow on the Hill and covert Catholicism would have been as evident to Jonson's audience as Banbury with Puritans', Pinciss explains, giving several examples of Harrow on the Hill's notoriety as a harbour for recusant Catholics.[123]

For Bartholomew Cokes, no distinct division separates the material from the immaterial, or flesh from spirit, as his attitude towards the puppets evinces. 'I am in love with the actors already', he exclaims, upon seeing them lying inert in Leatherhead's basket, and when Leatherhead reprimands him for '*handling*' a puppet, Cokes assures him, 'I will not hurt her, fellow. What, dost think me uncivil? I pray thee be not jealous. I am toward a wife', as if the puppet possessed the sense to feel assaulted (5.3.108, 5.4.3–4 sd, 5–6). Whereas Leggatt finds that Cokes lists people 'as junk' by clumping persons and objects indiscriminately in his recital of all that he has lost at the fair,[124] the reverse is true: Cokes elevates material objects to the level of the human, fastening on items as if they were living.[125] A typical and hilarious instance is when he cheers on his hobbyhorse as Puppet Dionysius scores a point against Busy in their dispute. (Before the argument interrupted the puppet show, Cokes was using his toys as puppets of the puppets, in effect, with the hobbyhorse designated as Dionysius [5.5.52]). Ian McAdam links Cokes's treatment of the puppets with Catholicism:

> the confusion between the literal and the figurative, the erroneous 'assumption that a visible sign is identical to the substantial thing itself ... is the fundamental error that the Protestants ascribe to the Roman Church'. No one shows this tendency so clearly in *Bartholomew Fair* as (the Catholic) Cokes, who fails to discriminate reality from illusion when he discusses the puppets in Leatherhead's basket, before the performance, as if they were actual living actors with performance histories.[126]

---

[122] Alison A. Chapman, 'Flaying Bartholomew', 511–41, argues that *Bartholomew Fair* satirizes Catholic practices, especially saints' legends and saints' plays, in a way that justifies Jonson's decision to renounce Catholicism and return to the Church of England in 1610.

[123] G.M. Pinciss, '*Bartholomew Fair* and Jonsonian Tolerance', 346–7.

[124] Leggatt, *English Renaissance Comedy*, 141.

[125] One reviewer even found something admirable about Cokes as played by Alan Howard in the Hands production – 'his gentle and touching recognition of the littleness of the puppets' (qtd in Jensen, *Ben Jonson's Comedies*, 48).

[126] Ian McAdam, 'Puritan Dialectic of Law and Grace', 426–7. McAdam is, in part, quoting Huston Diehl, *Staging Reform, Reforming the Stage*. Throughout 'Flaying Bartholomew', Chapman also discusses Cokes as a figure through whom Jonson relentlessly parodies distinctively Catholic practices.

In stark opposition to Cokes, 'a child, i'faith' (5.4.187), thrilled with every instrument, hobbyhorse, and gingerbread person he sees, the Puritan Busy insists on a rigid incompatibility between matter and spirit through his construction of the materials of the fair as false gods that ensnare and mislead the soul to its damnation. He denounces Leatherhead's toys as 'apocryphal wares', his hobbyhorse as 'a fierce and rank idol', his drum as 'the broken belly of the Beast', and Leatherhead himself as 'the proud Nebuchadnezzar of the Fair' for encouraging the worship of idols (3.6.48–52, 59–62). Similarly, Trash's gingerbread is a 'basket of popery', a 'nest' and 'idolatrous grove' of 'images', a 'flasket of idols', which must be (literally) overturned (64–5, 85–6). In destroying Trash's gingerbread before her eyes, Busy reacts more violently to her wares than to Leatherhead's. This reaction combines with his labelling of Ursula as 'Flesh' 'herself' and so 'above all to be avoided' as one of the ultimate 'enemies of man' (3.6.30–33), and with his projection of the 'disease' of carnal longing onto Win and women more generally. Busy's insistence on the opposition between the spirit and the flesh, in other words, involves a repeated (and as we have seen, both hypocritical and strategic) relegation of women to the negative side of this opposition. In contrast, Cokes, who has no concept of this division, also has no concept or ready means of constructing women as somehow weaker or inferior beings. His worst offence towards his fiançée, Grace (aside from his inability to perceive her strong disinclination to marry him), is his neglect of her when he becomes helplessly distracted by the fair's many novelties.

Obviously, we should see Cokes's and Busy's extreme views on the material objects of the fair as equally ridiculous. But while Cokes becomes a kind of unwitting 'martyr' for his faith (4.2.60), stripped of his possessions and even his outer garments just as the apostle from whom the fair takes its name was stripped of his skin,[127] in his harmless naïveté he is never converted to see things differently. Entirely forgetting his humiliation, Cokes is at his happiest at the puppet show, asking Leatherhead whether the puppets get 'flustered' and commenting that it would not cost much to feed them 'by reason of their littleness', despite Leatherhead's frank efforts to explain 'I am the mouth of 'em all!' (5.3.65–83). By contrast, Busy's less innocent view is the one most pointedly corrected at a climactic moment in the play.

Puppet Dionysius defeats Busy in their 'disputation' by demonstrating at once with the lifting of its garment that its animating 'spirit' is both physical and sexless. The puppet purports to prove to Busy through this gesture '*that I speak*

---

[127] Leatherhead refers to 'Saint Barthol'mew' at 5.1.1. This saint is often depicted holding his own flayed skin, perhaps most famously in Michelangelo's *The Last Judgment*. For a detailed account of the links between Bartholomew Cokes and Saint Bartholomew, a patron saint of the fair and its cloth-traders, skinners, and merchants, see Chapman's 'Flaying Bartholomew'. Marcus, *Politics of Mirth*, 58–9, also reveals the play's striking echoes of the liturgical texts read on the feast of Saint Bartholomew, which reflected on the limits of earthly authority.

by inspiration as well as he' (5.5.94–5).[128] Indeed, by revealing the physicality of its inspiration, Puppet Dionysius presents an image of the 'inspiration' that has moved Busy through the fair – an inspiration fully bound up with his physical longing for pig. Puppet Dionysius also demonstrates his ability to speak by the 'inspiration' of scripture as well as Busy, alluding to Saint Paul – a main source for ideas about the necessity of renouncing the flesh to live by the Spirit[129] – in his assertion that '*we* [puppets] *have neither male nor female amongst us*' (88–9).[130] With a biblical affirmation that gender is finally insignificant in matters of the spirit, this response to Busy's objection (and a conventional Puritan anti-theatrical objection) to cross-dressing on the stage not only undermines the objection, but also further challenges Busy's tendency to attribute to women weakness of spirit because of greater vulnerability to the body. But ultimately, the physical act of lifting the garments – the surprising material image before Busy and not the puppet's words – is what finally converts Busy to cease railing at the puppet show and 'become a beholder with you!' (100–101).[131] In a departure from his

---

[128] As Deborah Shuger, 'Hypocrites and Puppets in *Bartholomew Fair*', 70–73, asserts, Busy experiences a genuine, comprehensible conversion, precisely because the puppet's behaviour exemplifies the kind of hypocrisy, associated with role-playing, that animates Busy (along with Overdo).

[129] On the early modern (mis)appropriation of Paul's concepts of 'flesh' and 'spirit', refer to Osmond, *Mutual Accusation*, 10, 21.

[130] Puppet Dionysius is referring to Galatians 3:25–8.

[131] Alison Chapman, 'Flaying Bartholomew', insightfully reads Dionysius's surprising physical act as a parody of traditional accounts of martyrdom that claim the martyr's sacrifice converted the main persecutor. In particular, Dionysius's act alludes to Saint Bartholomew's martyrdom, which involved his skin being lifted to reveal a sexless body and purified soul beneath. As Chapman, 531–41, explains, 'the logistics of flaying entail removing the male genitals', and the more a martyr's body was destroyed the more his or her soul was considered sanctified in saints' legends. Whereas Chapman, 535–6, 539, reads Dionysius's gesture as undercutting the 'hagiographic view of flaying' by ultimately revealing 'nothing' of significance beneath the surface – that is, no purified, transcendent soul – I am arguing that the puppet's revelation does indeed mean something, both to Busy and in the context of the play as a whole. Nonetheless, tenets of Chapman's argument resonate with my contention that *Bartholomew Fair* denounces a hierarchical model of soul over body. She claims, for instance, that the play 'satirizes the idea that material, physical identity and sacred identity stand in inverse relationship so that as one is diminished the other is reinforced. In medieval hagiography, this formula holds, for the more the saints lose things or body parts, the greater their holiness becomes. For Cokes, however, losing the outward signs of his physical identity – his purses and his clothing – does not further identify him with Christ; it just makes him more of a cokes, which the *OED* defines as a "silly fellow, fool, ninny"' (536). From a different angle, then, Chapman sees the play as collapsing surface and depth, rather than treating body and soul as separate, antagonistic entities. For Chapman, 541, *Bartholomew Fair* shows that 'trying to get some transcendent human identity by piercing through or lifting off the surface is as futile as trying to skin a gingerbread man or a puppet (or even Cokes himself), for in the process of discovery,

own construction of poetry as the soul of a dramatic production, superior to the embodiment of costume, stage effects, and actors' bodies, here Jonson seems to be conceding the efficacy of material to instruct beyond words.[132] Indeed, the puppet chosen to confute the anti-theatricalist portrays not just Dionysius but *the ghost of* Dionysius in the motion (5.4.285). This detail draws attention to the most obvious instance on the stage – the representation of ghosts – of the necessary use of the material and the physical to convey and shape ideas about the immaterial or unseen.[133] Puppet Dionysius's garment-lifting compounds this point about the inextricability of spirit and material. In literally exposing its 'inspiration' and animating force, and in thus providing an image of the soul as implicated in the physical and beyond gender, Puppet Dionysius confirms the view, pervasive in the play, of the body and soul as mutually 'adulterated' for men and women alike.

Forwarding a notion of spirit and flesh as inextricable and equally imperfect from the start to oppose the conventional concept of the spirit as tainted and degraded by the flesh would seem an important tactic in defending the theatre from charges that it misleads and corrupts the spirit. Shershow has noted that Leatherhead, in filling the puppets with his voice, is a figure for Jonson as the 'mouth' of the actors of his play.[134] Leatherhead's decision to put Dionysius up as Busy's opponent is a decision to use a material, theatrical means to cure Busy's

---

you end up with nothing more than dry crumbs and stuffing'. This conclusion returns us to a view of the physical as somehow debased and inferior, with the spiritual as simply absent. My argument, in contrast, is that the play treats body and spirit alike with equal ambiguity. More than mere 'crumbs and stuffing', the body is irresistible and vibrant, as Ursula proves, while the wit, though sharp and amusing, can be cruel and pointless, as Quarlous demonstrates.

[132] The illuminating discussion in Thomas Cartelli, '*Bartholomew Fair* as Urban Arcadia', 171–2, of *Bartholomew Fair* as a saturnalian comedy that both critiques and owes a debt to the green worlds of Shakespearean romances includes a similar view of Jonson's comment on the didactic efficacy of theatricality. Cartelli suggests that Jonson could perhaps 'recognize (and expose) various images of himself in the trio of mystified demystifiers who define themselves in opposition to the puppet-monsters of invention embodied by the Fair and its unregenerate inhabitants ... [I]n reforming this trio ... [Jonson] may well be reforming himself as well: the "old" Jonson who, like the old Adam, sees enormity in every stone or pebble of human imperfection. At the very least, Jonson comes into a clarification of his own about ... the theatrical measures – puppets and all – a playwright may need to take to make his representation of reality both applicable and accessible to the workaday world around him'.

[133] The player's physical movement (does he walk lightly or seem to glide? quickly or slowly? restrict his motion or flit about the stage?) and voice (absent? hoarse or pained? altered from an earlier 'alive' appearance?), in addition to his garments (clanging armour? a thin shroud? the clothing he or she was murdered in? of light or dark colour?), would shape the concept of a ghost or disembodied soul (though as Hamlet's anxiety reminds us, these two immaterial entities are not always one and the same thing), for instance, in quite different ways.

[134] Shershow, *Puppets*, 102, 104, 106.

hypocrisy that proves effective when endless attempts to speak with him and punish him fail. This successful choice reflects on or justifies theatre's instructional role: stage behaviour can help to make a point or push towards a revelation not always possible or understood as words on paper or as oral lecture. Leatherhead even intimates the possibility that the material performance he is directing can convey a truth beyond his own knowledge: 'I am not well studied in these controversies between the hypocrites and us. But here's one of my motion, Puppet Dionysius, shall undertake [Busy], and I'll venture the cause on't' (5.5.28–30). That Puppet Dionysius plays not the drunken god of wine but a former tyrant and educator in the motion[135] further suggests how the material can dictate a truth or reality in a way that is impossible to ignore, forcing realizations when words fail. But the choice to frame an argument through the material inevitably involves relinquishing absolute authorial control over the message, allowing audience members to interpret for themselves, for instance, the reasons Puppet Dionysius's self-exposure effects such a change in Busy.[136]

In *Bartholomew Fair*, then, actual puppets expose the hypocrisy of attempting to puppet women on two levels: not only does Dionysius underline the absurdity of considering women to be more fleshly than men are, but even if this association were permitted to stand, the puppets, like Gloriana in *The Revenger's Tragedy*, also demonstrate the impossibility of fully controlling how the material signifies. Leatherhead might control the illusion of the puppets' insubordination when they beat him over the head at the slightest provocation, but he is quite unable to control how audience members, such as Cokes, for instance, read them, as indicated by his failure to disabuse Cokes of his belief that they are alive. Ursula shares with the

---

[135] For a discussion of Puppet Dionysius's literary antecedents and how they merge in *Bartholomew Fair*, refer to James E. Savage, *Ben Jonson's Basic Comic Characters*, 146.

[136] As Ostovich (ed.), *Bartholomew Fair*, 46, observes, here, and also when 'Overdo's oratorical attempt to mete out justice is silenced by his wife's vomiting', the 'frailty of the flesh defeats the word. The appeal to the senses overwhelms the appeal to the inadequate intellect'. Ostovich suggests that 'Jonson seems to be directing us towards a recognition of our world's failure to find a moral centre'. I would add as a further possibility that Jonson allows the physical an instructive role in morality through forcing recognition of the dishonesty of the intellect that assumes detachment from and superiority over the rest of humanity. In my position that Jonson relinquishes absolute authorial control in framing an argument through the material, I disagree with Shershow's position that 'the author pervades the mere performance from his position of inviolable externality: a sovereign voice whose presence transcends (and also requires) its own absence, a voice that reaffirms its own mastery in the apparent act of relinquishing it' (*Puppets*, 106). Cokes signals in the extreme the 'natural' response to the puppet as performative object – a fascination with the puppet itself that causes the audience to forget about Leatherhead, even if he is not concealed (he certainly pops up frequently to translate to Cokes and get beaten over the head by the puppets), let alone the puppet playwright, Littlewit, and final author, Jonson. For an alternative view on the play's relentless subversion of all forms of authority and its relinquishing of authorial control as not just an illusion, as Shershow claims, see Ch. 6 of Robert N. Watson, *Ben Jonson's Parodic Strategy*.

puppets a materiality that eludes definition or even firm categorization as material in opposition to spirit. While Winwife might derisively label Ursula 'an inspired vessel of kitchen-stuff' (2.5.70), out of all the play's characters, she is the most difficult to imagine as puppetable, not just because of her fiery temper, but also due to her sheer material unwieldiness. Winwife's is only one of several labels for Ursula tossed about by men in the play, demonstrating what Leggatt calls 'an itch to interpret Ursula, as though this will somehow bring her under control'. But, as Leggatt puts it, 'in the last analysis Ursula is Ursula, uncontrollably herself'.[137] When Mistresses Overdo and Littlewit emerge from Ursula's tent, some of Ursula's uncontrollability has rubbed off on them. Mistress Overdo, who has parroted her husband's sayings and invoked his authority repeatedly throughout the play, ends up silencing her husband by vomiting just as he is getting started on his indictment of everyone's 'enormities'. For Lori Schroeder Haslem, this moment is part of the play's overall construction of the female body as 'a locus of shame' in a way that the male body is not.[138] And yet the timing of Mistress Overdo's sickness also makes it a very visceral rejection of her husband's words of authority, which, until entering Ursula's domain, Mistress Overdo herself was verbally regurgitating. Likewise, only when Mistress Littlewit emerges from Ursula's tent does she cease to be her husband's puppet: she is no longer wearing the clothes Littlewit selected but is dressed as a prostitute instead. She neglects, moreover, to compliantly remove her mask despite her husband's frantic inquiries into her whereabouts. Granted, Mistress Littlewit's new attire poses new problems, suggesting that she has gone from being her husband's puppet to being Knockem's puppet. But it also shows Littlewit the consequences of treating his wife as property. Littlewit saw nothing wrong with displaying Win before his acquaintances and forcing her to kiss them when she didn't want to, but he is clearly uncomfortable when visually confronted with the implications of objectifying her for others' pleasure. Just as Puppet Dionysius's self-exposure silences Busy, and Mistress Overdo's physical statement puts an end to her husband's self-righteousness, Mistress Littlewit's physical change foils her husband's ever-ready wit – he has nothing more to say. Repeatedly, far from opposing the spiritual, the material instructs the spirit or mind much more effectively than words – and ignoring, dismissing, or presuming to control it can prove embarrassing or, in Vindice's case, fatal. Perhaps for Jonson an underlying message exists about the superior ability of the theatre, over the words of sermons (such as Busy's), to instruct, precisely *because* of the physicality that such sermons so often condemned.

---

[137] Leggatt, *English Renaissance Comedy*, 142.

[138] Lori Schroeder Haslem, 'Longings, Purgings, and the Maternal Body', 450.

Chapter 2
Tamer and Tamed

Women, Wit, and Will

That woman is not worthy of a soule
That has the soveraign power to rule her husband,
And gives her title up

— The Noble Gentleman (3.2.103–5)

A Womans humour hardly can Submit
To be a Slave to One she do's Out Wit

— Anonymous, 'Advice to Virgins'[1]

Maria, in John Fletcher's *The Tamer Tamed or, The Woman's Prize* (1609–1610?),[2] makes an explicit connection between her will and her soul when she first declares her intention to resist her husband's rule over her. In doing so, she recasts female resistance of male authority as a sign not of stubborn irrationality that only confirms women's need to be governed, but a sign of the intelligence and legitimate desire of the soul, that divine component of the self that scripture insists women and men alike possess. In his Shakespearean past, Petruchio[3] was clear about his project of quelling what Katharina called her 'spirit to resist' with the help of physical abuse in the forms of food and sleep deprivation (3.2.221). In Fletcher's play, Maria immediately closes off this avenue of power. By barring Petruccio's physical access to her body she ensures that the ensuing battle between them will take place on the grounds of wit. On this battleground, Maria proves superior to Petruccio, dominating him in a field formally reserved as the province of men: rhetoric – significantly, the art of influencing the *wills* of others.[4] Maria's rhetoric involves skilled reversals of Petruccio's misogynistic assumptions and former taming tactics in *Shrew*, reversals that carry implications for the social and ideological constructions of gender roles. Maria's central, most important reversal, as I will argue, inverts the associations of men with spirituality and rationality and of

---

[1]   Qtd in Kathleen Coyne Kelly and Marina Leslie (eds), *Menacing Virgins*, 19–20.

[2]   In Celia Daileader and Gary Taylor (eds), *The Tamer Tamed or, The Woman's Prize*, 8–9, the editors cite historical references indicating that the play 'cannot have been written earlier than the last months of 1609'. All references to the play cite this edition.

[3]   I follow the spellings of 'Petruchio' that the editions I am working with use. Thus, I refer to Fletcher's 'Petruccio' and Shakespeare's 'Petruchio'. References to Shakespeare's play cite *The Taming of the Shrew*, ed. David Bevington.

[4]   On the early modern view of rhetoric's influential power over the will, see Wayne A. Rebhorn, *Emperor of Men's Minds*, 15, and Neil Rhodes, *Power of Eloquence*, 25.

women with the body – a reversal that supports her claim to an intelligent will that merits recognition. The centrality of this reversal, however, does not necessitate that Maria reject the body or its role in rhetorical argument. On the contrary, Maria and her allies employ rhetoric that confuses the line between body and soul, and they supplement that rhetoric with pointed bodily gestures. In fact, insisting on having it both ways, that is, aligning women with the (superior) soul and men with the (inferior) body, and yet assigning positive value to women's bodies, is possible with rhetorical skill. In demonstrating this possibility, Fletcher's text ultimately exposes negative views of women's bodies and the association of women with bodies as themselves mere rhetorical constructs mobilized to subordinate women – rhetorical constructs that can easily be met with new ones more advantageous to women.

This chapter focuses on rhetorical debate over gender roles that invokes conceptions of the body-soul dynamic. Its concern with rhetoric moves away from Chapter 1's concern with material objects onstage that carried potential to undo basic distinctions between material and immaterial, body and soul, in ways that troubled misogynistic representations of women. As I will argue, Maria's rhetoric in *The Tamer Tamed* prompts a reconsideration of gender roles within marriage, both through its reliance on a sharp divide between soul and body and through its erasure of that divide at other moments. This chapter shares with Chapter 1, nonetheless, the argumentative premise that dramatic texts present a range of attitudes about the soul-body dynamic and that some of these attitudes open up space for more flexible, less misogynistic understandings of gendered relationships. I set up this chapter's discussion of rhetorical uses of the body-soul relationship in an onstage 'battle of the sexes' by first highlighting the significance of Maria's early insistence on a connection between her 'will' and her 'soul'. Second, I trace early modern understandings of the function and purpose of rhetoric that bear relevance to its use in Fletcher's play, and I review women's positions in relation to the study, practice, and definitions of rhetoric. Finally, I analyze in detail Maria's rhetoric of reversals and its implications for gender roles. This analysis will consider how Maria's eloquence, like that of other female characters, attends to and incorporates the body in her arguments without becoming a rhetoric *of* the body or retreating from the front of intellectual, verbal sparring. Of course, the rhetorical techniques I will be discussing are not new tactics and are certainly not unique to female characters. I posit, however, that staging women's appropriation of these techniques from a position of social subordination sharpens and changes their critical impact.

Will and Soul

The Tamer Tamed, Fletcher's revisiting of Shakespeare's *The Taming of the Shrew* (1592–1594), opens ominously for the widowed Petruccio's second wife, Maria. Sophocles and Tranio, gentlemen and friends of Petruccio, express 'pity' and 'fear' for the 'poor gentlewoman' whose father has 'dealt' 'exceedingly harshly, and not like a father, / To match her to this dragon' (1.1.8, 22, 5–7). Now that Petruccio is no longer 'the still Petruccio', having been 'forced' by his first wife's 'abundant stubbornness' to abandon his calm and calculated attempts to tame her and finally 'blow as high as she', even his friends acknowledge frankly that 'there is no safety' in being Petruccio's wife (37, 16–20, 29). Sophocles and Tranio rather coldly agree, in a sombre twist on the wagers that ended *Shrew*, that Maria, a 'tender soul', will likely soon be dead (40, 47–9).[5] In contrast to the men's passive observations about Maria's disposition, her cousin Bianca offers constructive advice, urging Maria to 'let not … / Your modesty and tenderness of spirit / Make you continual anvil to [Petruccio's] anger' (56–8).

Juxtaposed with these grim marital prospects, Maria's announcement that she will resist Petruccio's suffocating control[6] forswears any former 'tenderness' of 'soul' with exhilarating force:

> Adieu, all tenderness! …
> ....
> Mistake me not. I have a new soul in me,
> Made of a north wind, nothing but a tempest—
> And, like a tempest, shall it make all ruins
> Till I have run my will out. (73–9)

By resolving that before consummating her marriage her soul must storm[7] until her will is satisfied, Maria emphatically reinstates a claim that Katharina made before consummating her own marriage. Katharina insisted, albeit unsuccessfully, that she would not leave her wedding festivities 'till I please myself', observing that 'a woman may be made a fool / If she had not a spirit to resist' (3.3.80, 84, 92–3). Katharina comes to suspect that Petruchio, with his tactics of conditioning her to accept his governing will as substitute for her own, essentially attempts to hollow out her animating spirit in order to 'make a puppet' of her, an idea that I discussed in Chapter 1 (4.3.103). Maria credits Katharina's suspicion by expressing the link between spirit and will even more directly in her determination to avoid Katharina's fate. Maria's connection of spirit and will in her announcement of rebellion is not a fleeting or isolated reference. Revising Shakespeare's motif of the haggard in *Shrew*, Maria describes 'the free haggard' as 'that woman that has wing and knows it, Spirit and plume', and who, 'To show her freedom', will 'sail in every air / And look out every pleasure, not regarding / Lure nor quarry till her pitch command / What she desires' (1.2.151–7). Having 'spirit' translates here into acting in accordance with one's own will rather than stooping to obey another's.

---

[5]   Pamela Allen Brown, *Better a Shrew*, 141, even finds that the men 'hint strongly that Petruchio killed' his first wife, Kate.

[6]   Tranio tells us about how 'she must do nothing of herself, not eat, / Sleep, say "Sir, how do ye?", make her ready, piss, / Unless [Petruccio] bid her' (1.1.45–7).

[7]   For a contemporary etymology linking 'spirit' and 'soul' with 'breath', 'blast', and 'winde', see Simon Harward, *Discourse Concerning the Soule*, B1r–B2r.

Maria certainly emphasizes her refusal of Petruccio's will. She invokes Lucina, the goddess of childbirth, 'never' to grant her fertility nor aid with labour pains 'if I do / Give way unto my married husband's will' (108–13). She also vows to confront Petruccio even if he had the power to 'Cast his wives new again, like bells, to make 'em / Sound to his will' (168–70) – with the strong implication, of course, that he possesses no such power. Maria even confirms her resolve to Livia 'By the faith I have / In mine own noble will', designating her will as something sacred by which she can swear (137–8).[8]

The connection that Shakespeare's Katharina and Fletcher's Maria draw between the soul and the will is not a new one. A 1599 edition of John Davies's *Nosce Teipsum* lists the soul's 'powers' as '*life, motion, sense,* and *will,* and *wit*', claiming that the soul exercises the two latter powers without the body's assistance: 'Use of her bodies Organs she hath none, / When she doth use the powers of Wit and Will'.[9] In his 1604 *A Discourse of the Soule and Spirit of Man,* Simon Harward links soul and will when he clarifies that 'The Lord saith by *Ezekiel,* that he had given up the Israelites … to the soule, that is, the will and affections of them that hated them'. Harward's treatise notes Galen's reliance on Plato in his opinions on the soul, and reviews in detail Plato's standard division of the soul into three faculties, following Plato in his placement of the will as an 'appetitive' faculty serving a 'cognitive' faculty (the will desires what the mind and reason propound).[10] But, adding that 'some do more briefly bring it into a Dichotomy, making onely two parts of the soule, to witte understanding and will', Harward seems to add his own caveat concerning appetite (included in the will). He considers appetite to be 'a natural faculty of the soul' only when it obeys reason and natural instinct; when it refuses reason, the appetite is not so much part of the soul as 'a corruption' and 'infirmity'.[11] Writing almost three decades before Harward, John Woolton corrects what he perceives as the 'faltes' of Plato's explanation of the soul by insisting on a distinction between the 'Reasonable soul' and 'intellective sence'.[12] Woolton is clearly of the opinion, described by Harward, that the soul has 'onely two parts', claiming that the rational soul consists of the

---

[8]   Maria's claim that she will not 'lie' with Petruccio 'till I list' (1.3.109) finds an echo in Bianca's assertion that the 'whole country' cannot 'fetch' the women down 'unless we please to yield' (129–31), once again signalling that at stake in this battle is an acknowledgement and acceptance of women's independent wills.

[9]   John Davies, *Nosce Teipsum,* 12, 14. *Nosce Teipsum* went through at least four editions between 1599 and 1622.

[10]   Harward, *Discourse Concerning the Soule,* B3v, B4r–C1r, C4r. Harward does not limit his discussion of theories about the soul to Plato, but reviews the opinions of several Christian and classical philosophers on each topic about the soul that he covers.

[11]   Ibid., C4v.

[12]   John Woolton, *Immortalitie of the Soule,* fol. 9. For Woolton, Plato's main 'faltes' consist of labelling the functions of three body parts, the brain, heart, and liver, as three separate souls, and of confusing the actions of the soul with the actions of the brain or 'inner senses', which we share with 'beastes'.

'Mind understanding' and the 'Will'.[13] Drawing added attention to the association between soul and will, like Harward, Woolton also feels compelled to explain the crux about the will as part of the soul – the divine, immortal part of human beings – and yet capable of making wrong choices. Woolton's approach to this problem involves separating the soul and mind from the physical brain and bodily senses, arguing that the soul will only 'erre' in judgment if presented with misinformation, or 'false shewes and similitudes' which 'deceyveth the minde, simple and sincere in itself'.[14] Woolton pointedly sets his argument concerning the division of soul and brain 'agaynst' the opinion of physicians who posit that the soul's 'Actions' are 'impared' when the brain is 'distempered'.[15] Indeed, King James's physician, Helkiah Crooke, blurs the distinction so crucial to Woolton with his conviction that God's image could be found in both body and soul; nevertheless, he too aligns the will with the divine.[16] In his 1615 edition of *Mikrokosmographia* Crooke adapts Plato's tripartite structure of the soul to Christian doctrine by comparing the soul, which remains 'one' in 'substance' while containing 'three essential and distinct Faculties or powers, intellectual, sensitive, and vegetative', to the Trinity, also 'one in essence' yet 'distinct in persons'. Crooke reproduces the familiar division of the intellectual faculty (or rational soul) into 'Knowledge and Will', calling these 'two essential attributes resembling their prototype or originall in God'.[17] These examples offer differing interpretations of Plato, but together they illustrate the continuing notion of the will as one of the soul's highest functions, either paired with or serving 'reason', 'understanding', 'mind', or 'knowledge'.

Women and Rhetoric

Rhetoric, commonly defined as the art of persuasion, constituted an entire, fraught, and 'distinctive' discourse in early modern England.[18] The 'essential subject' of all works participating in this discourse is, in Wayne Rebhorn's summary, 'language (accompanied by supporting looks and gestures) as it is used to move people', or to

---

[13]   Ibid.

[14]   Ibid., fol. 10–11.

[15]   Ibid., fol. 10.

[16]   Helkiah Crooke, *Mikrokosmographia*, Preface to book 1, p. 2.

[17]   Ibid. Repeating his point about the soul's resemblance to the Trinity, Crooke later shifts his terms for the soul's faculties, but 'will' remains grouped with intellectual capacities and aligned with the divine: 'in [the soul] is a lively resemblance of the ineffable Trinity, represented by the three principall faculties, *Memorie, Understanding,* and *Will*' (book 1, Ch. 1, B2v).

[18]   Rebhorn, *Emperor of Men's Minds*, 2, see also 9–10, develops the argument that 'taken together, the hundreds of discussions of rhetoric produced during the Renaissance constitute a distinctive and recognizable *discourse*', a kind of 'specialized language' with its 'own distinctive lexicon of terms, its characteristic grammar, and its defining syntax of propositions and relationships'.

'affect people's basic beliefs and produce real action in the world'.[19] The practice of rhetoric aims to affect the will, in other words, and this understanding of its function will be important in light of the connection Maria makes between will and soul.[20] Given the power rhetoric was thought to have over the will, early modern descriptions of rhetoric unsurprisingly construct it (or refute this construction) as a kind of deceptive magic in some cases, able to produce a physical or almost physical force out of mere words.[21] Comparisons of rhetoric's effect to physical force, along with the location of gesture firmly within the province of rhetoric,[22] already begin to suggest that the practice and reception of rhetoric itself involved a disruption of the line between abstract thought and physical expression and impact. Maria and her companions, as I argue further on, make effective use of this quality of rhetoric in their stance against Petruccio and like-minded men.

Most women were debarred from formal training in rhetoric, which was closely tied to the study of Latin and prioritized in the education of boys from a range of social ranks.[23] Technical training in rhetoric was envisaged as the ideal preparation for a life of public service and political activities such as deliberating

---

[19]   Ibid., 3–4.

[20]   Ibid., 15, refers explicitly to rhetoric's effect on the will: 'when ... rhetoricians define the nature and function of the art in their treatises and handbooks, they stress its power above all else, specifically the power it puts in the hands of the orator to control the will and desire of the audience'. C.f. Rhodes, *Power of Eloquence*, 25: 'The ability to move – to affect the will – is the province of rhetoric', which, for Petrarch, meant that 'wisdom and virtue' were necessary to 'eloquence'.

[21]   Such constructions are not new to the early modern period, but take their cue from classical precedents. Refer to Rhodes, *Power of Eloquence*, 8–10, 19–20.

[22]   Cicero, whose influence on early modern thinking about rhetoric is, in the words of Rhodes, *Power of Eloquence*, 13, 'impossible to overestimate', places considerable importance on delivery, including the orator's use of voice, eyes, face, and gesture. For Cicero, *Ideal Orator*, 3.213, see also 214–23, 'delivery' is the 'dominant factor in oratory', and without effective delivery 'even the best orator cannot be of any account at all, while an average speaker equipped with this skill can often outdo the best orators'. Refer also to Rhodes, *Power of Eloquence*, 15–18, for a discussion of the perceived similarities between rhetoric and stage performance.

[23]   Rhodes, *Power of Eloquence*, 50, reports that 'by 1575', 'there were some 360 grammar schools in England'. This number meant that boys 'from relatively humble backgrounds, who would previously have had a minimal education, found themselves subjected to a quite extraordinarily intensive programme of verbal, rhetorical and literary training'. Jennifer Richards and Alison Thorne (eds), *Rhetoric, Women, and Politics*, 2, adopt a less optimistic view, noting that 'men of middle rank and above who attended grammar school or were tutored at home would have received at least a rudimentary introduction to the classical art of persuasion'. Rhodes and Richards and Thorne agree that 'few' girls had access to the study of Latin and rhetoric (Richards and Thorne, 2). Those who did were likely daughters of the nobility receiving instruction from a private tutor (Rhodes, 44).

in councils or at public assemblies, or pleading in courts of law.[24] As Jennifer Richards and Alison Thorne point out, since schooling in rhetoric was primarily training for skilled public oration, women's exclusion from public office and the perceived incompatibility between public speech and those qualities valued so highly in women, modesty and chastity, could be cited when male educators cared to justify rhetoric's omission from the instruction that girls received.[25]

Exclusion from technical schooling in rhetoric, however, did not prevent women from becoming competent rhetors. Technique was actually only part of rhetoric, and not the most important part, as Cicero makes clear in his *De Oratore* and Quintilian asserts in his *Institutio Oratoria*, both widely studied in the early modern period. Brian Vickers draws attention to illustrative passages in both to remind us that 'rhetoric, the art of persuasive communication, has long been recognized as the systematization of *natural* eloquence'.[26] While the term 'orator' designated an actual diplomatic profession, and humanists preferred to label themselves 'orators' instead of 'teachers', Rebhorn's affirmation that 'in a sense ... almost everyone in Renaissance society could have been dubbed an orator, and, what is more important, Renaissance people knew it',[27] resonates with the priority given to natural eloquence over its codification into a technique that really only strives to reproduce or emulate nature. Rebhorn explains that beyond law courts, official assemblies, and universities, the 'domain of rhetoric' could encompass 'courtship ..., confession and prayer, interventions aimed at the management of the family ..., and the advising and even occasional rebuking of

---

[24] Richards and Thorne, *Rhetoric, Women, and Politics*, 3. See also Rebhorn, *Emperor of Men's Minds*, 9, for the early modern view of rhetoric as 'a particularly political art'.

[25] Richards and Thorne, *Rhetoric, Women, and Politics*, 3–4. Girls' instruction, in contrast to the curriculum recommended for boys, usually aimed to prepare them to be competent in childcare, domestic chores, household management, and proper moral conduct for a wife, and therefore only necessitated the literacy skills necessary for tasks like record-keeping or reading 'the religious and homiletic texts that would fortify them against the perceived weaknesses of their sex'. See also Sara Mendelson and Patricia Crawford, *Women in Early Modern England*, 89–91, for a description of the content of girls' education.

[26] Brian Vickers, *In Defence of Rhetoric*, 1–2, emphasis added. In a passage from Cicero, qtd in Vickers, 1, just after outlining the 'main doctrines of rhetoric', one of Cicero's speakers asserts: 'the virtue in all these rules is, not that orators by following them have won a reputation for eloquence, but that certain persons have noted and collected the doings of men who were naturally eloquent: thus eloquence is not the offspring of the art, but the art of eloquence'. See Vickers, 1–3, for reference to a similar point in Quintilian and for further discussion of the priority assigned to 'natural' eloquence over the art of systematized technique. Early in *Ideal Orator*, 1.5, however, Cicero maintains that 'eloquence is founded upon the intellectual accomplishments of the most learned', as opposed to having 'nothing to do with the refinements of education' and depending solely on 'natural ability and practice'. See also Richards and Thorne, *Rhetoric, Women, and Politics*, 11, on 'ancient theoretician[s']' understanding of 'eloquence', the 'force, fluency or expressiveness of speech or writing', as 'pre-exist[ing] its codification as "rhetoric"'.

[27] Rebhorn, *Emperor of Men's Minds*, 6.

one's superiors'. In short, rhetoric 'could serve practically all individuals and fit practically all situations as it blithely crossed long-established boundaries among disciplines, professions, and social classes'.[28] Rebhorn does not include gender in this list of boundaries, but, given rhetoric's goal of influencing the wills of others and the difficulty of restricting it to men with technical training when natural eloquence trumps technique in importance, it certainly lends itself to challenging gender boundaries as well.

In *De Oratore*'s proposition that practice, not just theory, makes a good orator, Richards and Thorne perceive an opening for a feminist approach to early modern women's participation in the discourse of rhetoric.[29] They call on early modern scholars to foster greater awareness of the variety and possibilities of women's exercises in rhetoric by expanding our understanding of the term to include the study of eloquence as it develops from '"practice" in a variety of contexts' and not just from 'technical training and scholarly regimens', an adjustment that enables us 'to extend its exercise to women of all ranks'.[30] We might also elect for the term 'eloquence', as it opens up 'a vocabulary and a way of thinking that bring into view the often untutored persuasiveness of women's speech and its capacity for critical engagement with received ideas and structures of authority'.[31] Nonetheless, women were not always 'untutored', as Richards and Thorne are aware, since they could learn or gain familiarity with rhetorical strategy through other means, like attending plays; reading letters; listening to sermons; participating in litigation as witnesses, plaintiffs, or defendants; and taking part more generally and variously in oral culture.[32] These possibilities should not suggest that women's rhetorical power was limited to a combination of natural talent with the techniques that

---

[28]   Ibid.

[29]   Richards and Thorne, *Rhetoric, Women, and Politics*, 11. In particular, they point to a productive 'change of emphasis' in the possibility of 'appeal to Cicero's endorsement of practice-based rather than technical training in order to challenge the traditional authority of the schoolmaster', such as that found in Cambridge lecturer Gabriel Harvey's writing. Even if Harvey's discussion has in mind 'a community of university-educated male disputants', Richards and Thorne note that the 'importance he attaches to "practice" can be extended to include other kinds of speaker, other kinds of disputational context'. They go on to suggest that this possibility 'is already recognised in many of the handbooks and treatises that "theorise" restrictions on female speech, for these also reveal a more complex engagement with the practice of women's talk than is often taken account of in critical discussion'.

[30]   Ibid., 12. Richards and Thorne, 10, place the effort to expand the term 'rhetoric' in the feminist critical tradition which worked to productively expand the terms 'political' and 'public' from previous narrow constructions that neglected women's involvement in these spheres.

[31]   Ibid., 10.

[32]   Ibid., 12–13. Richards and Thorne suggest the first three possibilities and cite Laura Gowing's and Tim Stretton's findings on the 'intuitive grasp' of effective 'narrative strategies' evinced in testimonies from women who 'flocked to the consistory and equity courts in unprecedented numbers in this period'.

trickled down indirectly from men. Instead, women's 'gossip', a type of speech labelled as distinctly feminine, as Laura Gowing has shown, wielded power to define or destroy the reputations of both men and other women.[33]

Recognizing that Fletcher's portrayal of women besting men through a competent use of rhetoric does not belong innocuously to the realm of hypotheticals – just as scholars have recognized that *Tamer*'s portrayal of female insurrection alludes to very real women-led rebellions over enclosures and food shortages[34] – is important to appreciating the critical work the play is doing in terms of opening up alternative perspectives on gendered relationships. Showing female characters succeeding on grounds from which they are traditionally barred both challenges the basis for their exclusion and registers the real failure of such exclusion.

Fletcher's decision to foreground women's skill in rhetoric plays with gender assumptions on more than one level. The formal rhetoric most accessible to men was also subject to charges of being a negatively feminine practice. Just as misogynistic literature might berate women for bodily adornment or the use of cosmetics,[35] detractors of rhetoric attacked it as being concerned merely with the superficial decoration of language, and as working to (mis)guide the will by privileging technique, style, or a certain knack with words, over truth content, so that it was dangerously deceitful.[36] Opponents of rhetoric also discounted it as unstable because of its reliance on the passions – on stirring passions both

---

[33] See, for instance, Laura Gowing, 'Gender and the Language of Insult', 1–21, and *Domestic Dangers: Women, Words, and Sex*. In their work to complicate the term 'rhetoric', Richards and Thorne, *Rhetoric, Women, and Politics*, 10, seek to avoid the kind of oversimplification that defines rhetoric in opposition to 'feminised political talk – gossip, slander, conversation, etc.'.

[34] For a consideration of such revolts in connection with *Tamer* see Molly Easo Smith, 'John Fletcher's Response to the Gender Debate', 2–4; Fiona McNeill, 'Gynocentric London Spaces', 215–18; Daileader and Taylor (eds), *Tamer*, 8–9. For a historical account of women's rioting see Roger B. Manning, *Village Revolts*, 96–8, 115–16, 281. For Fletcher's country sympathies and sensitivity to the Midlands Revolt of 1607 see Gordon McMullan, *Politics of Unease*, 54–5.

[35] For more on early modern 'cosmetic culture' and on anti-cosmetic writings that address 'what was ... perceived as a feminine desire for physical beauty' (37), see Farah Karim-Cooper, *Cosmetics in Shakespearean and Renaissance Drama*, especially Ch. 2.

[36] Rebhorn, *Emperor of Men's Minds*, 9–10 and Ch. 3, investigates in detail how early modern rhetoricians struggle 'with the notion that rhetoric is, in some fundamental way, feminine'. He observes that even though rhetoricians defended rhetoric from the charge of being feminine by defining their art in '"masculine" terms as a matter of violent invasion and conquest', they could not resist 'imagining important aspects of their art in what their culture would have thought of as "feminine" terms such as procreation and bodily adornment' (16–17). Rhodes, *Power of Eloquence*, 8–19, traces opposition to rhetoric based on its deceptiveness from Plato's early objections into the Renaissance with writers like Stephen Gosson.

in the orator and in the audience.[37] Again, this means of discrediting rhetoric as an art is similar to the means of discrediting women for their supposed inability to control unruly passions, and thus legitimizing their subjection to men, who were purportedly more inherently reasonable beings, a problem I touched upon in Chapter 1. Women were excluded from formal training in rhetoric, but formal rhetoric was nonetheless attacked for being feminine. Rhetoric's proponents also appealed to misogynistic associations to instruct about proper technique. Tracing the 'narrative topos of overcoming a female enchantress or obstacle en route to completion and ending' in textual precedents such as the Bible, the *Odyssey*, and the *Aeneid* to make visible a connection between 'female figures and the extension or dilation of the text in order to defer its end or "point"', Patricia Parker has demonstrated a 'more specific link' between the female body and the 'rhetorical tradition of the dilation of discourse'.[38] Drawing on Erasmus's *De Copia*, Parker explains that the 'preoccupation of this massively influential text is not only how to expand a discourse ... but also how to control that expansion, to keep dilation from getting out of bounds'. This concern is reflected in 'countless Renaissance rhetorical handbooks which both teach their pupils how to amplify and repeatedly warn against the intimately related vice of "Excesse"'.[39] While dilation (amplification, expansion, and variation upon points), a part of rhetoric associated with the female body, was desirable, it was 'always something to be kept within the horizon of ending, mastery, and control'. A problematic association exists, in other words, between the need to master a woman's potentially unruly body and the necessity of controlling one's own potentially unruly rhetorical dilations.[40] When Fletcher portrays women's rhetoric as a tool for piercing through male deception and exposing, as opposed to enabling, unjust oppression, then, he reevaluates the negative associations between rhetoric and femininity, framing this link in a more positive light.

---

[37]   One of the speakers in Cicero's *De Oratore*, 2.185–96, for instance, discussing how to best move the emotions of jurors in favour of one's argument, recommends that orators pay attention to what emotions the audience brings to the case, and that they genuinely experience and express the emotions they wish to stir in their audiences (as opposed to pretending). For more information on early modern objections to rhetoric, refer to Rhodes, *Power of Eloquence*, 19, who connects the controversy over rhetoric to controversy over acting and poetry as part of the same continuing moral debate (Stephen Gosson, a staunch anti-theatricalist, for instance, also professed himself an enemy to rhetoric).

[38]   Patricia Parker, 'Literary Fat Ladies and the Generation of the Text', 253–5.

[39]   Ibid., 255.

[40]   Ibid., 255–6. For further cultural resonances of 'dilation' see also 256–8 and Parker's *Literary Fat Ladies: Rhetoric, Gender, Property*. For more on rhetorical dilation or *copia* see Rhodes, *Power of Eloquence*, 41–8. Rhodes, 59–63, also discusses how 'verbally elaborate styles began to be suspected of empty prolixity' in his discussion of 'rhetoric in crisis' at the beginning of the seventeenth century, when scholars such as Bacon advocated 'conciseness' over 'amplification', viewing such 'earlier rhetorical values as obstacles to the objective pursuit of truth'.

Fletcher was undoubtedly familiar with such conventions in rhetoric. Born into 'an overwhelmingly ecclesiastical family' and educated at Cambridge from age 11,[41] he probably received the education in rhetoric denied to most women. In *Tamer*, Fletcher takes what was already thought to be a tool potentially subversive of the status quo (in its aim of exercising power over the wills of others and its dependence on inherent skill more than on social position) and intensifies its subversiveness by portraying female characters adeptly employing it. He cleverly reveals how some of the most basic ways of thinking about rhetoric make this tool especially suitable to Maria's cause. A common way of imagining rhetoric, for instance, saw it as weaponry, and rhetorical debates as martial battles. Indeed, in Tudor education, as Rhodes points out, 'mastery of eloquence was clearly associated with development of masculine courage'.[42] Facing Petruccio's incessant threats of physical abuse, Maria is in need of weaponry. Wresting it away from its connection to exclusively male courage, she proves capable of wielding rhetoric effectively in order to actually, not just metaphorically, ward off threats to her person; for Maria rhetoric is a weapon, not in a school game but in a real struggle for her safety. The effect of the text highlighting rhetoric's potential to subvert traditional power relationships in this way is not to side with rhetoric's opponents, but to demonstrate the progressive social role that rhetoric could and should serve and to suggest the futility of attempting its suppression.

Maria's New Soul in *The Tamer Tamed*

I focus on Fletcher's *The Tamer Tamed* in this chapter primarily as an important contribution to stage representations of women that engage ideas about the body-soul relationship, and not to overlook or imply an absence of women's own rhetorical writings. My consideration here of Fletcher's representation of women recognizes, with Valerie Wayne, that 'polarization' between scholars focusing on woman-authored texts and those 'addressing feminist and other political questions concerning male-authored texts … misrepresents the ways in which ideological construction crosses biological boundaries'.[43] And yet actual women were not entirely absent from Fletcher's text if we follow Kathleen McLuskie, Alison Findlay, and Pamela Allen Brown in keeping in mind the important fact that women constituted a distinct and significant portion of the early modern audiences

---

[41] McMullan, *Politics of Unease*, 11.

[42] Rhodes, *Power of Eloquence*, 44. Rhodes continues, 'nearly all rhetoric books stress the importance of eloquence in the commandment of others, and a book such as Machiavelli's *The Art of War* acknowledges a similar relationship between military and rhetorical prowess'. See also Chapter 1 of Rebhorn's *Emperor of Men's Minds*, which discusses how 'writers tirelessly restate, albeit with their own emphases and for their own purposes, Cicero's and Quintilian's notion that rhetoric is a weapon' (9).

[43] Valerie Wayne, 'The Dearth of the Author', 222.

whose approval and patronage determined a playwright's financial success.[44] In particular, Brown's work on women and jesting culture defines a useful approach to considering women in the audience: 'listening for women's laughter', she proposes, 'forges an interpretive grid for resituating drama in relation to their desires and experiences. Women went to the theatre to hear plays that sometimes show signs of being tailored to appeal to their taste and judging wit'. *Tamer* could certainly be one of these plays, opening ample space for women's laughter.[45] At least one woman's 'judging wit' Fletcher might have had in mind was that of his patroness, Elizabeth (Stanley) Hastings, Countess of Huntingdon, with whom he enjoyed a 'close and relaxed (while nonetheless respectful) relationship', if his surviving letter to her is any indication.[46] If Fletcher sympathized with women he could, Celia Daileader and Gary Taylor claim, 'go boldly where no woman in 1610 dared to tread: on to a feminist stage'.[47] While the text itself, with its complex ideology, resists unreserved categorization as 'feminist', it does present female subject positions that push against conventional gender norms, and these subject positions link with dramatic play with the gendered soul-body dynamic.

---

[44]   Alison Findlay, *Feminist Perspective*, 4, see also 1–3, notes 'the tastes of female spectators had to be acknowledged and catered for by the companies whose productions they paid to see', and refers to Richard Levin's work on prologues and epilogues indicating that 'women spectators were thought of as a distinct constituency by those who worked in the theatre'. Brown, *Better a Shrew*, 31, draws on Kathleen McLuskie's work with her claim that 'a truly vital feminist criticism must be inclusive, and it must consider women not only as authors and performers but as audiences'. A passage she cites from McLuskie's 'Feminist Deconstruction' is worth repeating here: 'It is not enough to reject all literature of the past as the product of "male" culture or "male" critical traditions ... It is clearly not enough simply to privilege works by women writers, many of which are far from feminist in consciousness or tendency ... The strengths of a feminist criticism lie in its rejection of pre-existing meaning created by assuming an audience is male, and the process of deconstruction that inevitably ensues'.

[45]   Brown, *Better a Shrew*, 4. Brown, 140–44, also discusses *Tamer* in connection with her arguments on women and the culture of jest.

[46]   McMullan, *Politics of Unease*, 17. McMullan, 15, asserts that 'Fletcher was certainly part of the fifth earl's milieu by 1609', and Daileader and Taylor, *Tamer*, 8, claim that '*The Tamer Tamed* cannot have been written earlier than the last months of 1609'. On Elizabeth Stanley see also Daileader and Taylor, *Tamer*, 2–3.

[47]   Daileader and Taylor, *Tamer*, 1–3. Daileader and Taylor observe that Fletcher's own biography might furnish clues about his capacity to 'see the inhumanity' in 'traditional paradigms' such as wife-taming narratives, in that his lifestyle choices often went against patriarchal expectations. Fletcher never married, and Daileader and Taylor suggest that he therefore 'imagined' marriage, 'at its best, as a relationship between male collaborators: a "due equality" that requires and enables both parties "to love mutually" (5.4.97–8)'. And, 'whatever the truth, the relationship between [Fletcher and Beaumont] was so close that it was suspected of being sexual. Their alleged ménage-à-trois with a shared "wench" also scandalously violated the sanctities of monogamy'.

The juxtaposition of Petruccio's bets on his anticipated wedding-night sexual performance with Maria's proclamation that she has a 'new soul' is the first hint that Maria's and Petruccio's clashing ideas about women's bodies and souls will be central to their battle. With their first verbal sparring match Petruccio reveals fully the attitude that, in Maria's eyes, needs correcting. After threatening and pleading with Maria to come down from her fortified chamber and consummate their marriage, a publicly humiliated Petruccio unleashes a rant debasing women's bodies and utterly dismissing their minds. In this rant he equates Maria's very self with her sexual attractiveness, envisioning her turning into 'a thousand figures' to arouse him, and then imagining his response as an imperious rejection not just of her attempts, but of '*thee* and thy best allurings' (1.3.227–33, emphasis added). Once Petruccio reduces Maria to her body, he attributes the body's beauty to the intervention of male professionals such as the tailor and the doctor, without whose help women appear as 'flayed cats' (233–9).[48] He dismisses women's minds in a fleeting reference, likening them to women's 'not so handsome' bodies, except lacking the 'masks' of artificial beauty to hide their 'miserable' condition (235–9). Clearly Petruccio is clueless about Maria's conviction, as she expressed it to Livia just prior to setting up her barricade, that a 'woman' who 'lives prisoner to her husband's pleasure' has 'lost her making' and become a mere 'beast / Created for his use, not fellowship' (1.2.137–41).

In a move typical of her general strategy, Maria reverses the main points of Petruccio's attack. She begins by echoing words from his last sentence, as if signalling her project of rewriting Petruccio's perception of women, countering his 'And you appear like flayed cats' with 'And we appear – like her that sent us hither, / That only excellent and beauteous Nature' (1.3.240–41).[49] Maria makes no distinction here between mind and body as Petruccio does; in comparing women to 'Nature' she likens them to an abstract ideal, but an ideal that evokes concepts of physical, earthy beauty. Her description of women as 'too divine to handle' also mixes divinity with physicality (243). Rebutting Petruccio's construction of women's bodies as ugly without male intervention, Maria argues women are like 'gold, / In [their] own natures pure', and only 'blush like copper' once they 'suffer / the husband's stamp upon [them]' (243–7). For Maria, the moment of male interference with women's bodies, specifically through sexual intercourse, does nothing to improve them. Rather, this moment taints women's inherent beauty and divinity. Her metaphor of stamping for the change women undergo when they take

---

[48] Only 'doctor' is explicitly gendered male, but 'tailor' usually designates a male worker. The *OED*, 'tailor', 1a (emphasis added), notes that 'the "tailor" is the *man* who sews or makes up what the "cutter" has shaped', and provides examples of the title implying male gender. Petruccio's reference to 'the painter' in this same passage is more ambiguous. He is likely referring to women's practice of using makeup, but by grouping the 'painter' with the 'tailor', 'doctor', and 'silkworm', he frames painting, too, as something done *to* a woman, something for which she cannot claim credit.

[49] For a reading of the play's emphasis on the written word see Smith, 'John Fletcher's Response to the Gender Debate', 50–51.

a husband is fraught with cultural implications. She appropriates the conventional notion of women as naturally softer, moister, more malleable, and hence more passive creatures than men, wresting these qualities away from a construction of women's inferiority.[50] Maria aligns these qualities instead with purity and a superior nature or essence – like gold, more malleable but also more precious than a harder metal used to impress an image into gold or to mix with gold to form a harder alloy.[51]

The metaphor of stamping for sexual penetration, moreover, carries connotations of a man marking a woman as his property and imprinting his image upon her through the production of children.[52] Just as the sovereign's image stamped onto coin authorizes it as legitimate currency, through marriage a woman, in a sense, enters currency – following financial negotiations between her future husband and her father – to gain status in society as a matron.[53] Maria overturns such connotations by presenting the moment of rude 'stamping' not as a social elevation but as a personal debasement resulting from contamination with a man's already 'base' nature (she refers to men as 'alloys' even before they are 'mingled' with women [245–7]). Altogether, Maria's response focuses on an alignment of women with the divine and of men with an impure physicality that mars women's superior natures – a response that perhaps takes a jab at just how fixated on the physical Petruccio's defaming rant is.

Maria supports her claim that sex with men only tarnishes women's purity and divinity by treating as sacred the barricaded space that both preserves her virginity from Petruccio and serves as metaphor for her unstamped body. Livia must swear an oath and pass rigorous questioning before she can join the women in the upper room, and Bianca warns her in religious terms:

> If ye be false, repent, go home, and pray,
> And to the serious women of the city
> Confess yourself. Bring not a sin so heinous
> To load thy soul to this place. (2.1.85–8)

---

[50]   On early modern descriptions of women's physical constitution and its effect on their mental capabilities, see Michael Schoenfeldt, *Bodies and Selves*, 36; Lisa Perfetti (ed.), *Representation of Women's Emotions*, 4–5; Ian Maclean, 'Notion of Woman', 147.

[51]   C.f. Donne's explicit comparison of gold's purity and malleability with the soul in 'A Valediction: Forbidding Mourning'.

[52]   Wendy Wall, *Imprint of Gender*, 219, 346, discusses 'culturally widespread ideas about female impressionability' in relation to the printing press. Entering print was a sexualized act, since 'to be "pressed", as Renaissance texts suggest, is to "play the ladies part", to undergo the "press" of the male body during sexual intercourse'. Maria's metaphor of sexual intercourse as an imprinting or stamping of gold is closely related.

[53]   Mendelson and Crawford, *Women in Early Modern England*, 131, note that wedlock 'elevated women to a loftier rank in village as well as elite society', with matrons, for instance, sitting 'together' in Church, 'in front of their single counterparts, to mark their higher standing in the community'.

Once satisfied with Livia's sincerity, Maria instructs her to 'fling ... away' any 'fond obedience ye have living in you / Or duty to a man, before you enter', as ''twill but defile our off'rings' (120–22), again underscoring the idea that Livia is setting foot on hallowed ground. Elsewhere, Maria, Bianca, and their allies appropriate military terminology to describe their battle with the men: in warning Livia of the punishment of treason;[54] in their talk of 'parley', 'the foe', 'treaty' and 'conditions', 'strengths' and 'forces' (2.1.15, 75, 2.4.2,4, 2.5.93, 117); in one Country Wife's vision of a 'glorious fall' in battle, that would see her buried 'with her distaff' (rather than sword) 'stuck by me, / For the eternal trophy of my conquests' (95–100); in their assumption of titles such as 'soldiers' and 'Joan of Gaunt' (2.5.164, 96); and so on.[55] These military references simultaneously communicate the seriousness of the women's resolve to battle for their 'cause' while poking fun at the pretentiousness of a field considered the province of men.[56] Maria's and Livia's use of religious language works in much the same way, by referencing an institution often exclusive of and oppressive towards women while also imagining a religion in which women are the priestesses, confessors, and only practitioners. They do not suppress the body, but fully include its free expression through rebellious merry-making in this quasi-sacred, upper-chamber space, likely the stage's balcony. The balcony fortress appropriately presents a visual image that supports the theme of 'woman on top' and the notion that women are closer to the divine, since we see them looking down at the men, who call 'up' from below.[57] Maria's chamber is at once 'the play's inner sanctum', as Daileader

---

[54] Bianca promises Livia that 'if we do credit you / And find you tripping', she will suffer a fate worse than the assassin of 'the Prince of Orange', who suffered dismemberment and disembowelment alive before being decapitated and quartered, a standard punishment for treason (as Daileader and Taylor observe in their note 44–5).

[55] A City Wife also conveys the seriousness of the women's resolve by telling the men that if the women give up on their cause the men can 'degrade us of all our ancient chambering', 'hew off' the 'symbols of our secrecy, silk stockings', 'our petticoats of arms / Tear off', and 'our bodkins break / Over our coward heads' (2.5.105–10). As with the substitution of distaff for sword, here the City Wife lists traditional places and signs of women's authority in a way that references military practice and weapons, with playful puns on 'coat of arms', and on 'bodkin' as both 'dagger' and 'hairpin'. The Country Wife adds to this a reference to women's 'plackets' as 'crests' (112).

[56] In Theatre Erindale's production (2009), the three county wenches who confer briefly to give us an idea of the women's forces gathering in support of Maria creep stealthily onstage from three different directions and find one another by using secret bird calls. The bird calls, along with the women's armour and weapons (they brandished kitchen utensils such as rolling pins, ladles, and pot lids, and one wore a colander helmet), won laughter from the audience. Their appearance effectively conveyed the creativity and spirited sense of humour of the women's contingent, without detracting from a sense of their resolve and capability.

[57] For a discussion of 'the long tradition of "women on top" available to Fletcher and his audience from common culture', see Brown, *Better a Shrew*, 141, and Natalie Zemon Davis, 'Women on Top', 156–85.

puts it, and a 'sanctuary for [the women's] own pleasure'. She likens the chamber to Ursula's booth in *Bartholomew Fair*, which, 'however profane' as a space for 'riotously physical activities', also contains 'a certain mystery'.[58] In troubling the line between spiritual and profane, soul and body, Maria troubles Petruccio's rhetoric as it depends upon a view of the body as debased and a view of women as base for being so caught up with the body.

Maria's prolonged virginity contributes to this liminal position that she emphasizes between body and soul, and suggests how this liminality threatens male authority. By extending the period of her virginity indefinitely beyond the wedding ceremony, Maria creates and occupies a threshold between maid and wife, effectively defying patriarchal categorization of women according to their marital status.[59] In a spiritual invocation that centres upon her body, Maria asks the goddess Lucina to 'never unlock the treasure of my womb' until she has made Petruccio 'easy as a child' (1.2.108–14).[60] Lucina is closely associated with Diana, who formed part of the triple Diana or triple Hecate, a goddess 'concerned with the life of women', whose multiple aspects could be appealed to for help in areas such as fertility or childbirth problems, vengeance, and magic.[61] Enlisting Lucina's aid, then, Maria taps into the literary motif of the magic power of virginity, a motif Milton is still making use of in 1634 with his Ludlow masque *Comus*. This masque features a lady's decisive defeat of the carnally tempting Comus with her 'rapt spirits' kindled to a 'flame of sacred vehemence' in defence of the worth of

---

[58]   Celia Daileader, *Eroticism on the Renaissance Stage*, 55, 67.

[59]   Kelly and Leslie, *Menacing Virgins*, 21, describe an increasingly common early modern view of virginity as 'a temporary stage through which a young girl passed on the way to chaste marriage' and as 'a valuable commodity but with limited shelf-life'. Maria reclaims control over this 'commodity' traded between fathers and prospective husbands and de-naturalizes virginity as a stage that both enables and ends with marriage. Kelly and Leslie add, however, that 'to chart the history of virginity as a steady evolutionary progression from a religious ideal in the Middle Ages toward a more secularized ideal in the Renaissance would obscure the extreme instability of the concept of chastity in both periods. Medieval and Renaissance attitudes toward virginity are not generalizable and evolutionary but specific, changeable, and often conflicted, yet it is clear that virginity's signifying force is no way annulled by contradictions'. 'Virginity's signifying force' in early modern England is itself a complex topic of wide scope, though it is not central to my current discussion. For further studies of early modern stage representations of virginity, apart from the concentration on Elizabeth I's 'virginal politics' which has tended to dominate such study according to Kelly and Leslie (18), refer to Regina Buccola and Lisa Hopkins (eds), *Marian Moments*, and Marie Loughlin, *Hymeneutics*. The latter explores the topic through a focus on Fletcher, examining his 'characteristic' emphasis on 'sexual violence' and the 'female virginal body' in light of the close connection in many of Fletcher's plays between the 'politics of body and of state' (22–3).

[60]   This was a powerful moment onstage in the Theatre Erindale's production, with Maria advancing towards the audience to hold her arms out and gaze upwards intensely as she called to Lucina.

[61]   Mark P.O. Morford and Robert J. Lenardon, *Classical Mythology*, 208–10 and 638.

her virginity.[62] The lady is only fully released from the grip of Comus's venomous gums of glutinous heat by a magical virgin's ritual cure: the nymph Sabrina touches these gums with 'chaste palms moist and cold' and sprinkles drops from her pure fountain on the lady's breast, fingertip, and 'rubied lip' (911–19). Just as the masque presents virginity as the source of a supernatural, conquering power (albeit represented in very physical terms through Sabrina), the choice to remain a virgin, which Maria adopts for 'ten, or twenty' nights, 'or say a hundred, / Or indeed till I list' (1.3.108–9), was often a choice of bodily governance intended to attain and signify special spiritual status. Pre-Reformation English women had the option of entering convent life as brides of Christ, for instance, and their physical abstinence could translate into considerable spiritual and mental liberty. As Kathleen Coyne Kelly and Marina Leslie note, during the Henrican Reformation 'fear of women sequestered together running their own affairs contributed to arguments for disbanding what had become centers of female autonomy and learning'. Kelly and Leslie find that 'in the Renaissance, virginity continued to be equated with sacred as well as secular capital'.[63] Maria's decision to extend her virginity certainly arouses fear in Petruccio, as his concern not just for his lust but for his 'reputation' evinces (2.5.9). And in her own way Maria certainly uses physical abstinence to secure spiritual and mental liberty, in that before Petruccio can 'have me / As you would have me' he must submit to her will (4.1.152–3).

Maria also uses her physical abstinence as a pause, disrupting male control over her body's transition from virgin to non-virgin, in order to demand proper recognition of the power, both physical and non-physical, that women wield in childbearing and -rearing. When Petruccio voices his expectation that Maria have 'a noble care / Of what I have brought you and of what I am / And what our name may be' (3.3.106–8), Maria asserts her power over, not obligation towards, Petruccio's name and status, telling him 'that's in my making', with the explanation that:

> ... there was never man – without our moulding,
> Without our stamp upon him, and our justice –
> Left anything three ages after him
> Good and his own. (108–13)

Maria revisits and again revises, here, the sexual metaphor of stamping. Sophocles, too, adds to the stamping metaphor by discreetly advising Petruccio to concede temporarily to Maria's demands from her guarded fortress, since 'When ye are once a-bed, all / these conditions / Lie under your own seal' (2.5.149–50). Sophocles's reference to the document seal as an image for consummation recalls

---

[62] John Milton, *A Masque ... Presented at Ludlow Castle*, 793–9. Further references to the masque cite this edition.

[63] Kelly and Leslie, *Menacing Virgins*, 20, 17–18.

the legal precedence of a husband's official seal over that of his wife.[64] Insinuating that as soon as Maria is 'under' Petruccio during sex she will be under his power, Sophocles also alludes to the legal practice of coverture, which subsumed a married woman's legal identity under her husband's.[65] In her return to this stamping imagery, however, Maria places men in the position of soft material amenable to 'moulding' and receptive of 'stamping', with women as the moulders and stampers. 'Moulding' might refer to the shaping of a child within the womb, which was thought to be affected by the mother's imagination.[66] It could equally refer to a mother's moulding of her children's characters as she raises them, a process that could begin with nursing, since children were thought to absorb the moral qualities of their mother (or wet-nurse) through her breast milk.[67] Maria's talk of 'moulding', then, cites women's creative powers of 'making' without designating these powers as strictly physical or spiritual. Instead, the two are inextricable in the processes the word evokes. In the context of women's creative powers, Maria's claim that no man is left anything good 'three ages after him' without women's 'stamp' and 'justice' suggests that the only lasting legacy a man can hope to leave behind are his children; that all men and their offspring necessarily bear the 'stamp' or image of their mothers; and that women's discretion or 'justice' ultimately controls children's 'legitimacy' or even their very existence.[68] These implications resonate with Maria's conviction that Petruccio, who has grown too boastful a 'breaker of wild women', needs a reminder of his origins, and her consequent determination to 'Turn him and bend him as I list, and mould him / Into a babe again' (1.2.171, 174–5).

Petruccio himself weighs in on the stamping metaphor with an extreme articulation of the very view that Maria opposes when she troubles the soul-body distinction and aligns women with the divine: the view that women are inferior

---

[64]   Brigitte Miriam Bedos-Rezak, 'Seals and Sigillography', 732, records that 'by the mid-thirteenth century a regression in [high-ranking women's] seal usage had occurred, so that they sealed thereafter only in concert with their fathers, husbands, and sons, and only those *acta* involving their own property ... Quite often, documents issued in the name of both spouses were authorized by the seal of the husband alone'. While 'gentry and non-noble women seem to have had a more independent use of their seals', it seems their freedom became curtailed with marriage: 'if unmarried, they sealed deeds in their own names; if married, they sealed ... deeds conjointly with their husbands'.

[65]   On 'the implications of the doctrine of coverture' see Mendelson and Crawford, *Women in Early Modern England*, 36–7. 'Common law', they note, 'made a sharp distinction between single and married women, treating marriage as the norm: all women were either "married or to be married". Man and wife were one person, and that person was the husband'.

[66]   Ibid., 28. See also Ian Maclean, *Renaissance Notion of Woman*, 3.7.5.

[67]   Mendelson and Crawford, *Women in Early Modern England*, 29.

[68]   Indeed, when Maria delivers her hilarious eulogy for Petruccio when he fakes death, she applauds herself for being a 'careful woman' who, 'born only to preserve' Petruccio, 'Denied him means to raise' any children, 'Out of the fear his ruins might outlive him / In some bad issue' (5.4.36–9).

to men because they are more bodily than men. 'Then, and never / Till then', he retorts, referring to Maria's initial mention of women being stamped by men, 'are women to be spoken of, / For till that time you have no souls, I take it' (1.3.247–9).[69] References to the belief that women lack souls emerge in several seventeenth-century texts, especially in those treating questions about the origin of the soul. John Davies's *Nosce Teipsum*, for instance, lists among the 'erroneous opinions' of the soul's creation the idea that God locks up 'virgin spirits' in 'a *secret cloister*' 'untill their mariage day',[70] an idea that resonates with Petruccio's claim that women receive their souls during sex. Davies clarifies a few stanzas later that no precedent exists for claiming a woman's soul comes from her husband, since the Bible is clear on the detail that when God took Eve from Adam's rib, 'Doubtlesse himselfe inspir'd her soule alone: / For tis not sayd, he did mans soule divide, / But tooke flesh of his flesh, bone of his bone'.[71] Harward repeats Davies's point when he, too, observes that no biblical reference exists stating that God took 'soule from [Adam's] soule' along with bone of his bone.[72] Even if

---

[69] Daileader and Taylor footnote this speech as registering 'a position seriously maintained by some Christian theologians'. The earliest English reference to the theological argument that women were soulless, according to Percy C.H. Herford and Evelyn Simpson, *Ben Jonson*, 464, n. 370, appears in *Mary Magdalene* (1567), when Infidelity argues with Mary. Simpson also refers to sixteenth-century disputes over whether women possessed souls, the Ambrose commentaries on St Paul, and *Mary Magdalene* in *A Study of the Prose Works of John Donne*, 141–2. Mendelson and Crawford, *Women in Early Modern England*, 62, briefly discuss the idea that women had no souls as a 'proverb or "common saying"' in 'plebeian settings', besides noting its currency as an 'academic joke'. See also the overview, in Maclean, *Renaissance Notion of Woman*, 2.4.1–2.4.3 and 2.5.1, of theological and philosophical sources for the debate on whether 'woman' is a 'human being' and on whether 'woman' is 'made in the image of God'.

[70] Davies, *Nosce Teipsum*, 26–7.

[71] Ibid., 30.

[72] Harward, *Discourse Concerning the Soule*, VI. F1v–F2r. Harward blames the mistaken notion that women gain their souls from men – one of the 'gross heresies' he tells us Augustine warns against – on the importance Tertullian attaches to the biblical description of God inspiring a soul into Adam, juxtaposed with the lack of any mention about God doing the same for Eve at her creation. Harward simply dismisses Tertullian's argument by stating the needlessness of narrating the same point twice. Using much the same terms as Harward, William Hill, *Infancie of the Soule*, D2r, C2r, also faults Tertullian as a source for the position that Eve's soul derived from Adam, and actually credits the soul with determining an infant's sex, for 'he is not a Man or Woman, before the soule be united unto the Body'. Of interest in Hill, D2r, E2r, is his refreshing attribution of authority to women on the issue of whether or not unborn infants have souls. Hill cites women's experience of an infant moving in the womb to demonstrate the presence of the soul, and interestingly, he refers to the biblical story of John leaping for joy in Elizabeth's womb and the infant John's expression of a passion (joy) to prove the presence of the 'rational' soul in the infant. His willingness to appeal to women's experience as authoritative evidence, however, falls apart when Hill explains that we can trust the words of Elizabeth and Mary during their meeting because undoubtedly John and Christ were speaking *through* these women, as if using their mothers as conduits for holy writ.

the position that men endowed women with souls through intercourse was most often invoked to be discounted,[73] it is clearly a recognizable stance with its own logic, and one that Petruccio is familiar with. That it is a position often discredited does not make it any less available for Petruccio's use. In fact, texts that cite, explain the sources of, and then discount this belief paradoxically perpetuate it as a recognizable opinion. Petruccio's immediate, retaliatory jeer that virgin women are soulless, an effort to save face before his peers by devaluing Maria's humanity, further evinces that women's souls and what they might represent are centrally at issue in the gender power struggle between Maria and Petruccio. His appeal to the notion of women's soullessness, of course, also helps the audience to further discredit Petruccio's overall behaviour as extreme and erroneous.

In suggesting that a woman lacks a soul and thus significance prior to consummating marriage with a man, Petruccio attempts to deny Maria her personal autonomy along the same lines that, as Lynette McGrath has shown, early modern culture more generally obstructed women's 'access to a legitimate sense of self' by aligning the 'self' with the 'soul' and gendering that soul as masculine in contrast to a feminized body.[74] As I touched on in Chapter 1, McGrath finds that women writers overcome this cultural inhibition through 'invest[ing] a positive sense of self in their very physicality' or through departing altogether from 'the "male mind"-"female body" dichotomy by insisting on the interconnected functions of women's minds and bodies in intellectual activity'.[75] But with Maria, Fletcher imagines a woman constantly changing her position, sometimes troubling and at other times maintaining a conceptual distinction between soul and body. Regardless of intention, Fletcher's play thus gets at the problem that women writers constructing their subjectivity faced in having to grapple with and respond creatively to dominant ideology's alignment of women with the body. His portrayal of Maria highlights how differing and dynamic models of the body-soul relationship could be mobilized as rhetorical constructs in ways that subordinate women to men – and in turn, in ways that reject such subordination.

A refusal to recognize a division between body and soul can prove as debilitating and oppressive to women as their relegation to one 'side' of the divide. Consider the example of Shakespeare's Lucrece, who has internalized the cultural association of bodily chastity with spiritual integrity to the extent that she resolves to destroy

---

[73]   If the idea that Eve had her soul from Adam was often discounted, the notion that infants' souls – or at least their 'divine' sparks of life – were imparted through the father and not through the mother, while also contested, finds expression later on in the writings of prominent medical authority William Harvey, as Eve Keller, *Generating Bodies and Gendered Selves*, 112–15, discusses. For further references to (and an exciting rejection of) Adam as the source of Eve's soul and the implications of this view, see also Woolton, *Immortalitie of the Soule*, fol. 21 & 27, and Henry Woolnor, *True Originall of the Soule*, 33, 49, 203–113 (it should be 203–14, but at what should be page 209 the page number reads 109 and the succeeding pages count from 109).

[74]   Lynette McGrath, *Subjectivity and Women's Poetry*, 47.

[75]   Ibid., 47, 64.

her violated body as the only means to free her 'pure mind' from contamination in a 'polluted prison'.[76] Dekker, Rowley, and Ford's Mother Sawyer in *The Witch of Edmonton* suffers accusations about the state of her soul that are grounded solely on her physical appearance. She knows that her neighbours label her a witch and assume she has sold her soul to the devil, only because her body is elderly, gaunt, and stooped.[77] In England, many women were executed for having engaged their souls in traffic with the devil based on the evidence of bodily markings supposedly indicating where demonic familiars sucked the witch's blood.[78] We could also claim that Shakespeare's Petruchio recognizes an 'indissoluble connection'[79] between Kate's spirit and body when he sets out deliberately to subdue her spirit by weakening her body.[80]

In response to Petruccio's physical violence Maria twice reiterates the body-soul distinction she first insisted upon with her wedding-night barricade that forced her new husband to engage with her wit without recourse to her body. Petruccio has a revealing story for Sophocles when his friend suggests that Maria may have only refused sex with Petruccio when they finally shared their first night together because 'Some women love to struggle' and Petruccio should have tried 'a little violence' (3.3.7–9). 'She had it', Petruccio assures him, but it only caused Maria to vow that without her consent, he 'might take her body prisoner, / But as for her mind or appetite –' (9–15). An exchange very similar to this one occurs in a powerful moment onstage. Petruccio, exasperated at how successfully Maria turned his feigned illness against him – a ploy he designed to shame Maria for her treatment of him – tells her that she merits being beaten 'as much as may be', that her actions practically 'cry "Come beat me"' (4.1.127, 140–42). Maria's forceful response to this threat of battery echoes her response to Petruccio's threat of marital rape. She promises that 'the first stroke' Petruccio dares will drive her to 'turn utterly' from him 'for ever' (142–8). In both scenarios Maria makes clear

---

[76] William Shakespeare, *The Rape of Lucrece*, ll. 1653–9, 1701–29.

[77] Thomas Dekker, John Ford, and William Rowley, *The Witch of Edmonton*, 2.1.3–8.

[78] Keith Thomas, *Religion and the Decline of Magic*, 445–6.

[79] McGrath, *Subjectivity and Women's Poetry*, 74, n. 44.

[80] Lisa Hopkins, *Female Hero*, 12–14, also perceives negative consequences of the view of women's 'physical and mental operations' as 'never far apart', 'indeed … intrinsically linked'. Hopkins notes that following Fallopius's discovery of the fallopian tubes in 1562 'medical writing increasingly presented woman, especially in her procreative capacity, as not the inverse of man, but his physical and temperamental opposite pole, and women's bodies thus increasingly become a favoured arena for medical investigation … and provide the dominant discourse for describing their mental as well as their physical processes. Increasingly, then, bodies, and in particular motherhood, or at least the biological ability to be a mother, become perceived as both the defining characteristic of women and as the means of their pathologisation and indeed criminalization'. See also Maclean's chapter on 'Medicine, Anatomy, Physiology' in *Renaissance Notion of Woman* on the link drawn between women's physiology and their supposed lesser mental faculties, especially 3.3.9 and 3.7.4.

to Petruccio that overpowering her body does not amount to enjoying control over her person; in fact, exerting physical force over Maria entails permanently losing access to her 'mind' and 'appetite' (usually located in the soul). Evincing Maria's progress in her cause, a baffled Petruccio withholds his fists to instead hurl an angry wish, only after Maria's exit, for 'witchcrafts, herbs, or potions' that 'can again unlove me' (4.1.157–9). Maria is bringing Petruccio to realize that an admiration of her 'wit', a 'something / Certain' he 'married for' (25–6), is incompatible with his urge to dominate her body.

Maria's tendency to shift between maintaining and blurring the line between body and soul constitutes a rhetorical strategy that contributes to her mastery of her husband's old taming tricks, a mastery that itself evinces her soul as the seat of her intellect. Maria's refusal to consummate her marriage constitutes a sophisticated reference to one of the old Petruchio's tactics. Reasoning that Katharina will become amenable to his will when 'passing empty' and physically weak (4.1.190), *Shrew*'s Petruchio deprives Katharina of food and sleep. Maria, in turn, resorts to 'fasting' Petruccio until he recognizes her will (1.2.96), although she deprives him only of herself. Where Petruchio relies on physical coercion, Maria's taming strategy prompts Petruccio to rationally weigh a choice between satisfying his urges elsewhere or hearing her out, and she correctly wagers that Petruccio will not find her replaceable with another woman's body nor risk losing her sharp and interesting mind.

Maria's method of fasting her husband is only the first of many taming techniques that she successfully appropriates. She controls all of her entrances and exits,[81] as when, after warning Petruccio (in the above example) of what he can expect if he strikes her and outlining expectations for his future behaviour, Maria ends with an abrupt 'And so farewell for this time' before turning heels on him (4.1.156). In this assertive exit she presents a pointed contrast to Shakespeare's Kate, whose exits and entrances are noticeably under Petruchio's control after her marriage, as when he hurries her offstage, away from her own wedding festivities unwillingly; permits her to return to Padua for Bianca's wedding only when satisfied with her readiness to affirm his every word; and commands her to return onstage for a demonstration of her obedience as part of the play's final bet, and then to exit and re-enter, bringing the other wives. Conversely, in *Tamer*, Petruccio is the one whose entrances and exits are controlled. He is locked against his will into his own home under Maria's pretence that he suffers from the plague, only managing to burst out, gun in hand, after everyone else has left. In the Theatre Erindale's production, a raging Petruccio erupts onto centre stage through clouds of smoke with the flash and crack of gunshot. These stage effects, juxtaposed with Petruccio's disappointment that no one remains to witness his fierce display (his first words upon storming onstage are 'Are ye all gone?' 3.5.95), convey perfectly the futility of his male bravado. Later, when Petruccio lies about plans to embark

---

[81]   See Daileader, *Eroticism on the Renaissance Stage*, 57–8, for a related discussion of Maria's seizure of control over space.

on a long voyage, really intending 'nothing less' and only aiming to further 'try' Maria, she goes along with his ruse, enthusiastically hurrying him on his way with a comical offer of a ready-made packed lunch and advising him not to miss the next tide (4.4.184–5, 198–9). Maria does not exit when Petruccio instructs her to 'Get thee going', threatening to 'kick thee to thy chamber' (210–12). Instead, she stays to make a joke of Petruccio under the guise of solicitation for his best interests, commending him for undertaking travels to mend the 'flying fames here of your follies, / Your gambols, and ill breeding of your youth' (216–18). Interrupting Petruccio's parting curse to redirect it towards Petruccio himself, Maria again exits on her own terms, leaving Petruccio with no choice but to head to the docks to conceal his bluff. Maria even ruins Petruccio's carefully planned re-entrance in a coffin when he feigns death from his marital misery in a last-ditch effort to shame Maria. Rather than responding with remorse as Petruccio expects, Maria reflects (most hilariously) on the blessing of Petruccio dying before he could heap more dishonour onto his name, effectively forcing Petruccio's real and humiliating entrance when he springs from his coffin in despair. Adopting Petruchio's former trick in *Shrew* of signalling his control over Kate by directing her entrances and exits, Maria demonstrates that this ability is not a male's prerogative.

Maria challenges and overrides Petruccio's credibility in the scenarios surrounding his controlled entrances and exits, turning another of Shakespeare's Petruchio's methods against him. In *Shrew*, Petruchio successfully pits his word against Kate's in public when he explains away her fierce rejection of him in her vow to 'see [Petruchio] hang'd' before she weds him, assuring the company that

> 'Tis bargain'd 'twixt us twain, being alone,
> That she shall still be curst in company.
> I tell you 'tis incredible to believe
> How much she loves me. (2.1.304–7)

Maria more than matches this move when, elaborating on a cue Petruccio himself provides by pretending to be gravely ill, she turns his illness into the dreaded plague. She easily convinces the guard to forcibly quarantine him and all of his acquaintance to flee his presence, all while Petruccio desperately protests that he is 'as sound, / As well, as wholesome, and as sensible / As any of ye all' (3.5.55–7). The approach of pitting 'my word against yours', of discrediting an opponent's words while bolstering one's own credibility, is part of a contest of wills that plays out, in both plays, through the 'tamer' imposing on the 'tamee' an alternate version of reality. Petruchio forces Kate to bend to his words as if they constituted her reality when he insists that it will be what time he says it is before they travel to her sister's wedding, that the sun is really the moon, and that Vincentio is a young maiden. Maria adopts Petruchio's old approach when she constructs her own version of the events surrounding her husband's pretend sickness. Within Petruccio's hearing, she puzzles about why he would 'Not let his wife come near him in his sickness' while taking two old women to be his keepers, as if deeply hurt by this. In *Shrew*, Petruchio tests Kate's submission by having her affirm his words even when they are blatantly false, and thus risks appearing as ridiculous as she does; to onlookers they come across as playing a strange game in calling things their opposites.[82] Maria outdoes Petruccio by inventing a story of her husband's 'sickness' that allows for her self-presentation as an innocent, admirable, and wronged wife while attaching scandal to Petruccio with the suggestion of his preference for elderly matrons. The plausibility of the version of reality that Maria imposes on Petruccio[83] departs from the absurdity of Petruchio's claims in *Shrew*, a difference that lays claim to the very real power of women's speech or 'gossip' to make or destroy men's reputations within a community.[84] In keeping with her opening declaration, Maria's will overpowers Petruccio's, demonstrating the strength of her 'new soul' with its storming wit.

Just as strategic as Maria's 'gossip', her bodily carousing and gesturing move beyond unruly behaviour, signifying a rejection of male authority to respond intelligently to yet another of Shakespeare's Petruchio's past taming techniques. Petruchio's 'mad attire' and behaviour at his wedding (*Shrew*, 3.2.124), along with Biondello's account of the diseased mount Petruchio rides to the ceremony, have been likened to a skimmington ritual that Petruchio himself performs.

---

[82]   When Petruchio halts travel to Bianca's wedding upon being contradicted by Kate, Hortensio does not lecture her to learn obedience to her husband, but advises her to simply 'Say as [Petruccio] says or we shall never go', that is, to at least superficially comply in the interest of practicality (4.5.11). Taking Hortensio's counsel, Kate's new 'compliance' with Petruchio registers his absurdity and sounds rather like an exasperated concession to a fool with whom she is simply tired of fighting when she tells him he can call the sun a 'rush candle' if he pleases and that 'the moon changes even as your mind', but that she will go along with it so long as they can continue on their way (4.5.12–22). Petruchio himself first addresses Vincentio as a 'gentle mistress' to test whether Kate will follow his lead, and Vincentio addresses both 'fair sir' and 'merry mistress' when declaring how 'your strange encounter much amaz'd me' (27–54).

[83]   When alone with Petruccio, Maria is just as direct as Shakespeare's Petruchio is about making her spouse conform to her words:

> What I have said
> About your foolish sickness, ere you have me
> As you would have me, you shall swear is certain,
> And challenge any man that dares deny it,
> And in all companies approve my actions. (4.1.151–5)

[84]   As Brown, *Better a Shrew*, 145, observes, 'The resolution [of Petruccio and Maria's stand-off] is brought about by liberal applications of social pressure through threats of gossip and loss of male honor. As one of Petruchio's friends puts it: "Now you must grant conditions or the Kingdom / Will have no other talke but this" (2.4.84–5)'. McNeill, 'Gynocentric London Spaces', 219–20, gives an account of how Petruccio betrays his awareness of and anxiety over 'female intelligence networks' in his urgent desire to 'contain the labyrinth of secret female passages that lead through the city'. For the power of women's gossip to determine social reputations, see also Laura Gowing, 'Gender and the Language of Insult' and *Domestic Dangers*.

In order to avoid the potential shame of being married to a scold, 'Petruchio seizes control of the community's most threatening weapon' of humiliation.[85] While skimmingtons shamed husbands who could not properly harness their wives, in Petruchio's hands the skimmington humiliates and dishonours Kate on her wedding day. Shakespeare's Petruchio continues this mad behaviour by railing at and beating his servants, and, in short, out-shrewing Kate, 'kill[ing] her in her own humor' (4.1.85, 180). In Fletcher's play, when Maria is 'i'th'*flaunt*' with the women, dancing with 'their coats tucked up to their bare breeches' and 'firk[ing] it / In wondrous ways' with a 'stick of fiddles' (2.5.35–7), she simply matches her new husband's behaviour when he boasts of his sexual prowess by taking bets on his ensuing performance, thus 'killing' him 'in his own humor'. She responds even more directly to Shakespeare's Petruchio's use of his body to humiliate Kate as well as to preempt and avoid, by parodying, as Larue Love Sloan argues convincingly, the shaming ritual the community could potentially put him through, by similarly using her body against her new husband. Just when Petruccio is about to 'vex' Maria by feigning an intention to undertake extensive travel, he receives word that she is 'mad':

> As mad as heart can wish, sir. She has dressed herself
> (Saving Your Worship's reverence) just i'th' cut
> Of one of those that multiply i'th' suburbs
> For single money, and as dirtily.
> If any speak to her, first she whistles,
> And then begins her compass with her fingers,
> And points to what she would have. (4.4.45–51)

Pedro parenthetically apologizes for the blunt information that Maria is dressed like a prostitute, suggesting an awareness of how Maria's behaviour inevitably reflects onto Petruccio. Besides drawing negative attention to Petruccio just as Shakespeare's Petruchio did to Kate, Maria also willingly exposes herself to the public, here in a guise considered shameful and earning her similar suspicions of madness. She, too, circumvents by appropriating and outdoing the kind of social shaming the community might impose on her, which, for unsubmissive women, usually centred on some form of humiliating public display, such as being carted or wearing a scold's bridle. If the diseased, stumbling, unkempt horse that Shakespeare's madly dressed Petruchio reportedly rides to his wedding is Petruchio's way of representing and distancing himself from what disorderly marriage looks like, the horse a detailed 'caricature of an impudent wife',[86]

---

[85]   Larue Love Sloan, 'Caparisoned like the horse', par. 8.

[86]   Ibid., 10. I am paraphrasing Sloan's argument, which is more intricate and thorough than I have space to recapitulate here. Sloan explains how the mount in skimmington processions was understood to represent the unruly wife, the rider the henpecked, incompetent husband, and analyzes in fascinating detail the cultural and historical implications of every aspect of Petruchio's horse and his own attire.

then what does Maria's equally deliberate appearance as a prostitute say about Petruccio and her marriage to him? If Shakespeare's Petruchio can demonstrate the unattractiveness of a marriage in which a wife refuses to submit to her husband, Maria demonstrates her vision of a marriage in which a husband objectifies his wife as his property, acquired for his use and pleasure and bound to obey him. Maria's refusal to speak during her display except by 'tokens' might preempt or parody the punishment of the scold's bridle that she could expect as an outspoken woman, but it also underscores her comment on objectification and turns Petruccio's earlier injunction of silence ('If you talk more, / I am angry, very angry' [1.2.168–9]) against him.

Maria's rhetoric, then, uses both her wit and her body to trump Petruccio's wit. The Theatre Erindale's version of *Tamer* interpreted the 'signs and tokens' with which Maria responds to Petruccio when dressed as a prostitute as a dance that perhaps referenced flamenco, with twirling punctuated by tambourine clapping and pointed stomping. The effect was to emphasize her ability to communicate through her body in a way that both baffled Petruccio and made clear to the audience a sense of confidence and authority. In response to Maria's provocative and unsettling bodily display, Petruccio can only talk himself into a trap: he babbles on in the face of Maria's silence, which she only breaks when he finally mentions travelling, to hurry him on that voyage he has no intention of making.

Maria proves she is more than the intellectual match for her husband's former, triumphant, Shakespearean self, mastering point by point his boasted taming techniques.[87] She thus fulfils the rhetorical principle of 'invention', assiduously gathering her material from a 'received bank of wisdom' or 'storehouse of examples' culled from her husband's past behaviour rather than from formal rhetorical training.[88] More radically, men in general have supplied a 'storehouse of examples', as Bianca suggests in her encouraging words for Maria:

---

[87]   Smith, 'John Fletcher's Response to the Gender Debate', 39, also sees Fletcher's play as a 'pervasive commentary' on *Shrew*, a 'calculated intertextual glance' that 'comments, rewrites, and undermines the ideological assumptions in Shakespeare's' play. Similarly, Margaret Maurer, 'Constering Bianca', 186–206, perceives a 'deeply conceited connection' between the two plays, and her argument that Fletcher was attentive to a particular construction of Shakespeare's Bianca that critics have tended to overlook demonstrates just how detailed Fletcher's revisiting of Shakespeare's text could be.

[88]   'Invention' is the first part of rhetoric for Cicero, *Ideal Orator*, 1.17–18, and a basic principle of 'invention' is the accumulation of knowledge: 'To begin with, one must acquire knowledge of a very great number of things, for without this a ready flow of words is empty and ridiculous; ... Moreover, one must know the whole past with its storehouse of examples and precedents'. Rhodes, *Power of Eloquence*, 14, explains that 'invention' is less associated with 'originality' than it is today, and more with 'having at one's disposal a vast bank of received wisdom' to draw from. In place of the 'storehouse of examples' at a male scholar's fingertips, Maria substitutes 'examples' from the education she and other women have received from men, both anticipating Petruccio's moves based on 'precedents' from his life with Katharina as well as from other husbands' treatment of their wives, and turning Petruccio's own 'examples' against him.

> All the several wrongs
> Done by imperious husbands to their wives
> These thousand years and upwards, strengthen thee!
> Thou hast a brave cause. (1.2.123–6)[89]

By portraying Maria as methodically taking on and besting Shakespeare's Petruchio in each of his witty manoeuvres, Fletcher's play suggests that social advancement or triumph over one's adversaries through the skilled exercise of eloquence is not the prerogative of men solely. Through showcasing rhetorical skill at the service of female characters vying for equality with men, Fletcher restores rhetoric to its usefulness as a subversive, rather than oppressive and exclusive, social tool (subversive here of traditional gender, rather than class, hierarchy). And the play's presentation of Maria's struggle as exemplary of a more general struggle all women face, along with the epilogue's direct appeal to women and men in the audience to take home the play's message about gender equality within marriage,[90] extends this subversiveness beyond the world of the play, beyond an intertextual conversation between Fletcher and Shakespeare.

Fletcher's portrayal of women rhetors also troubles a gender stereotype built into constructions of rhetoric itself, namely, the link that Patricia Parker demonstrates between the female body and the 'rhetorical tradition' of 'dilation'.[91] One of several contexts for the idea of dilation that Parker identifies is the 'putting off of coitus or consummation … a purportedly female plot in which holding a suitor at a distance creates the tension of a space between as well as an intervening time'.[92] Parker's recognition of this plot in *A Midsummer Night's Dream* could also describe *The Tamer Tamed*:

> the erotic consummation promised in the play's opening scene is deferred for a time and space which coincides with that of the play as a whole and which is achieved only when a 'partition' or wall associated both with the hymen and with the rhetorical 'partition of discourse' is finally put 'down'.[93]

---

[89] McMullan, *Politics of Unease*, 159, documents how, as in this example, 'again and again, Byancha acts to escalate the subversiveness of Maria's pronouncements by moving away from a focus upon the individual to a general assertion of women's rights'.

[90] Anna Bayman and George Southcombe, 'Shrews in Pamphlets and Plays', 20, note that the epilogue, likely given by Maria, may have been a later addition. David Wootton, '*The Tamer Tamed*, or None Shall Have Prizes', 206–25, stresses the complexity and ambiguity of early modern understandings of 'equality', drawing on contemporary uses of the word. Wootton cautions that the existence of two very different definitions of equality should prevent us from interpreting the play as a straightforwardly proto-feminist text. He argues that while the ambiguity behind the 'equality' the play promotes certainly allows for audience members to take away a more progressive, proto-feminist interpretation, it also gives Fletcher space to reassert male authority.

[91] Parker, 'Literary Fat Ladies', 253–5.

[92] Ibid., 258.

[93] Ibid., 259.

Although it seems to fit this pattern, Fletcher's play actually alters a pervasive way of thinking that Parker alerts us to: the rhetorical handbook's exhortation to keep within bounds the technique of dilation as it is associated with the female body, and the closely related narrative topos of conquering or stripping the female enchantress in order to 'penetrate a text's meaning' and reach the desired ending.[94]

Maria delays the text's ending through the simultaneous delay of bodily penetration, but in her decision to 'protract' the 'offerings' of 'Hymen' she seeks not to defer a resolution (1.2.95–6); rather, she actively brings about a resolution that would otherwise never occur. In response to her sister's advice that she 'Divest [herself] with obedient hands: to bed' (1.2.101), Maria is unambiguous about the purpose of 'dilating' the marital narrative in between ceremony and consummation:

> To bed? No, Livia. There are comets hang
> Prodigious over that yet. There's a fellow
> Must yet, before I know that heat ...
> Be made a man, for yet he is a monster. (102–6)

Petruccio, not Maria, is the occasion of the dilation, the obstacle that must be overcome, the 'monster' that must be conquered before the narrative can properly end. To prove the seriousness of her resolve to tame Petruccio, Maria asks the goddess Lucina, 'when I kiss [Petruccio], till I have my will, / May I be barren of delights', framing Petruccio's bad behaviour as an impediment to *her* sexual pleasure that she must deal with in order to enjoy him (1.2.120–21). The description of Petruccio as 'monster', moreover, speaks to the construction of the female enchantress as monstrous beneath the surface, as Spenser's Duessa exemplifies, whose 'misshaped parts' are catalogued in the narration of how she is finally 'despoild' by Arthur and Redcrosse.[95] Petruccio envisions Maria suffering the shame of a similar public stripping when she has led everyone to believe he was plague-infected: 'The blessing of her grandam Eve light on her! / Nothing but thin fig leaves, to hide her knavery!' (3.5.75–6). Despite this vindictive wish, Petruccio himself is the one who undergoes repeated and humiliating exposures at Maria's hands.

Maria exposes the 'dragon' within Petruccio that Tranio warns of in the first few words of the play (1.1.7). Simply by maintaining her resolve to 'dilate' on her marriage narrative, Maria reveals how quickly Petruccio can shift from a sugary 'Why, who offends you? / I come not to use violence', to, before the end of the same scene, swearing to 'devil' the women 'By these ten bones', to 'starve' or 'fire' them out, and to force them to beg mercy 'on their bare knees' (1.3.103–4, 84, 274, 279–88). Maria later exposes before Sophocles the same insincerity and impulse towards violence in Petruccio. She sets up this revelation

---

94   Ibid., 253–5.
95   Edmund Spenser, *The Faerie Queene*, I.viii.46–8. See Parker, 'Literary Fat Ladies', especially 252–5.

by soliciting Sophocles's opinion (while ignoring Petruccio) about purchases for her new residence, even flirting with him to increase Petruccio's annoyance. When Maria finally directs angry attention at Petruccio upon his demand of 'obedience' from her, Sophocles attempts to intervene on his friend's behalf, asking Maria to 'understand him' (3.3.113). Maria claims she understands him only too well to be 'most spiteful' and 'sooner fire than powder', upon which Petruccio quickly loses his temper, threatening to 'drag' Maria to her 'duty' (114–26). 'Drag me!' Maria exclaims, underlining the violence in this response, and Petruccio immediately changes his tone, insisting 'but I am friends again' (26–7). At this about-face Maria slyly remarks, 'Now you perceive him, Sophocles' (128). Just prior to this outburst, Petruccio had tried to mollify his demand for 'obedience' by explaining that he did not 'urge' it by 'way of duty' but 'of love and credit', but here, Maria reveals beyond all question the falseness of such protestations by provoking a demonstration of the rage always bubbling just beneath their surface. By drawing Sophocles's attention to Petruccio's abrupt shifts in tone, Maria makes explicit that, through her entire interaction with the men, she is making a point.

Later, Maria draws forth another revealing response from Petruccio in order to make a point of defying it: his infuriated threat to beat her for convincing everyone he had the plague. Maria cries and seems to reply meekly as Petruccio unleashes a string of insults,[96] until he speaks of physical abuse as the only just response to her past behaviour. The possibility that Maria feigns tears to encourage Petruccio's belief that he is for once enjoying a position of dominance finds support in the fact that Maria does not cry at any other moment in the play in which she endures similar insults and threats. At Petruccio's threat of battery she stops her tears instantly, moreover, to launch a powerful speech of defiance that maintains every word of 'what I have said / About your foolish sickness' and repeats her earlier insistence that Petruccio confess to having wronged her by faking illness. The only other time Maria cries occurs during Petruccio's most humiliating exposure and at a crescendo of Maria's wit. In this later instance, Maria exposes publicly Petruccio's shameful fakery of his own death by weeping not with grief over losing him, but, hilariously, with thankfulness at the blessing of his death before he could commit more folly. Only with the final exposure of Petruccio springing from the coffin, at a loss for words and lacking, for once, a violent, aggressive response, can the narrative finally find resolution. Maria's treatment of Petruccio reverses completely the familiar motif of the female monster who must be unveiled for the resolution and ending of a narrative to occur. And while Maria's ensuing promise to cease her 'tricks' and become Petruccio's willing 'servant' might seem like a giant step backwards to embrace patriarchal ideology (5.4.46, 52), it really signals her complete confidence in her victory and in the unveiled Petruccio's transformation (indeed, she must even reassure Petruccio that he need

---

[96] See, for instance, 4.1.108–9: '*Petruccio.* Thou most poor, paltry, spiteful whore – do you cry? / I'll make you roar, before I leave. / *Maria.* Your pleasure', and 126: '*Petruccio.* Well, go thy ways. *Maria.* [*Going*] Yes'.

not fear her). Far from capitulating under pressure, Maria generously extends an olive branch at the play's end. She chooses to soften Petruccio's defeat by showing that she can play the demure wife as well as the defiant one, but only after making clear that her will and intelligence determine her behaviour towards him, not a concession to male authority. Even Petruccio recognizes the choice involved when he swears he will never give her 'cause' to resume her opposition (53–4).

Even aside from these exposures, Petruccio, not Maria, is associated with the negatively 'feminine' practice of rhetorical dilation. Apart from conspiratorial conversation with Bianca and Livia, Maria does not reveal her plots to the audience through monologues before we witness her publicly acting upon them. Petruccio, by contrast, is a weak rhetor who cannot control the length or direction of his own speeches. Upon breaking free from his quarantined quarters, for instance, Petruccio claims he 'would now rip up, from the primitive cuckold, / All [women's] arch villainies' except 'that I should be thought mad, if I railed' (3.5.98–101). He then disregards his own warning about the connection between ranting and madness to 'rail' on women for the next 30 lines, providing a 'catalogue' of their evil ways (102–31). Such rants from Petruccio betray unruly, irrational (and thus supposedly more bodily) passions, like rage.

In exposing Petruccio's penchant for violent outbursts Maria essentially exposes to what extent his authority as husband depends upon physical coercion and how little it has to do with reason.[97] Petruccio's incessant rants and threats of physical abuse, in other words, combined with their main cause – his frustration at not being able to satisfy his bodily urges – associate Petruccio strongly with the body.[98] Maria, too, brings emotions into her rhetoric, but she employs them more

---

[97] Indeed, Petruccio is so fixated on the physical from the beginning that when Maria first rebels on their wedding day, he cannot imagine it would be for anything but material gains and so assures Maria that he possesses adequate 'means', 'conditions', and 'fortunes' for her physical comfort, and even 'that mettle / A man should have to keep a woman waking' (1.3.139–49). Maria prods him to think differently by insisting that 'the ends I aim at' are not such 'idle outward things' (149–52). She then charges him by something intangible, that 'duty or respect / To me from you again that's very near / Or full the same with mine', to 'go to bed and leave me / And trouble me no longer … / For know, I am not for you' (1.3.199–209). Instead of complying in demonstration of that 'duty', Petruccio remains mired in the physical with his appallingly violent threats, including promises to beat Maria so severely with cudgels she will be bedridden; to confine her to a hard, uncomfortable bed to increase her pain; to make her sit on an uncomfortable wooden apparatus of punishment; to force her to eat food which will obstruct her stool for a year, etc. (1.3.279, 287–8, 2.3.20–23, 28–32).

[98] Fletcher bolsters the association between men and the body (as base and vulgar) that he sets up through Petruccio with the aged Moroso, who cannot stop obsessing about having sex with Bianca even though she might be young enough to be his granddaughter; with the men surrounding Petruccio and Moroso, who make vulgar jokes about Moroso's sexual prowess and about the bodies of Maria's female allies (Jacques is especially forthcoming with such jokes); and with Petronius, who is as eager and insistent about cudgelling Maria as Petruccio is. Instead of neatly countering this association by aligning women entirely

effectively as tools under her manage, as when she stuns Petruccio with her abrupt shift from tears to angry defiance. Maria's anger is effective (stopping Petruccio in his tracks when he proposes to beat her) and controlled (she directs anger at Petruccio in response to something he has just said, and exits before her speech turns into a rant or Petruccio has a chance to respond). Conversely, Petruccio's anger is ineffective and out of control. He shamefully tries to retract his rash statements and cannot prevent himself from venting at length to the audience when Maria is not even present. In this contrast, Maria's anger resembles what Gwynne Kennedy has called 'just' or legitimate anger, spurring one to noble or righteous action – the type of anger normally attributed to men – while women's anger, which Petruccio exemplifies, was often discredited as irrational, rash, and under the unstable influence of the body.[99] Nonetheless, Maria does not shun the place of emotion in rhetoric altogether; she is just more emotionally savvy. In this sense, Fletcher draws on the strong cultural association between women and emotion, and rhetoric's reliance on an understanding of emotion, to suggest women's potential to be the best rhetors.[100] In light of rhetoric's aim of controlling the wills of others as a means of self-empowerment, this suggestion presents social equality as – at least theoretically – within women's reach, while also getting at the heart of gender hierarchy as a social construct and not a natural order based on any inherent lack in women's intelligence.

If women were supposedly more susceptible to the passions because of their greater vulnerability to bodily influences, they were also, according to Laurent Joubert's *Treatise on Laughter* (1579), 'more inclined to laughter than men because they "engender much good blood"'.[101] As with the ability to navigate the passions, the ability to elicit laughter proves to be a strength in the art of persuasion. Maria is not only at her wittiest during the speech that seals her victory and pushes Petruccio to his final exposure; she is also at her funniest, which highlights the importance of laughter in her rhetoric. Maria turns Petruccio's last effort to publicly shame her into a sophisticated and skilfully performed joke. Petruccio's fake death at first seems to have the effect he would desire. Pedro and Jacques want to 'Hang' Maria, 'Split her!' 'Drown her directly!' 'Starve her!' '[Shit] upon her!' and 'Stone her to death' (5.3.58–60). Maria's father confronts her with Petruccio's body, admonishing her before onlookers for killing a man that was 'too good for ye' with 'Your stubborn and unworthy way' (5.4.4–5). Again, Maria's response is to weep, but when her tears are met with the men's

---

with the mind, as we have seen, Fletcher's Maria includes the body in her rhetoric in a way that, rather than degrading her wit or legitimacy, reconstructs or elevates the body, setting it quite apart from the base and vulgar.

[99] Gwynne Kennedy, *Just Anger*, especially 1–20.

[100] On women's bodiliness and consequent increased susceptibility to emotions in comparison with men, see Schoenfeldt, *Bodies and Selves*, 36; Perfetti, *Representation of Women's Emotions*, 4–5; Maclean, 'Notion of Woman', 147; McGrath, *Subjectivity and Women's Poetry*, 40.

[101] Brown, *Better a Shrew*, 28.

approval, she cautions them to 'judge me as I am, not as you covet' (12), before launching into a delightfully comical eulogy that, while shattering their expectations, is in perfect keeping with Maria's character. Maria's show of emotion is far from the sign of weakness that Petronius and Sophocles want to take it for. Instead, it is a powerful mode of expression entirely under her control, at the service of her quick wit. Indeed, Maria's bid for laughter in her speech depends upon the audience's appreciation of the irony in her words and the cleverness of presenting her tears – which the men expect to be tears of remorse – as tears of pity and thankfulness. Maria pities 'How far below a man' Petruccio was. She is thankful that 'He had a happy turn; he died' before having 'begot more follies', and that she had enough foresight not to let him reproduce foolish offspring (24, 27, 30).

Livia gives an equally funny and witty speech as she is poised to triumph over the alliance between her aged suitor and her father by marrying Roland, her own choice of husband. Under guise of serious apology to Moroso while pretending to be on her deathbed (pulling off Petruccio's trick, only with more cause and with more success), Livia delivers an absolutely hilarious recapitulation of how she 'abused' Moroso. She recounts how she gave him 'purging comfits / at a great christening once, / that spoiled his camlet breeches', and how she strewed a stairway with peas so that Moroso, 'ev'n with his reverent head ... / told two-and-twenty stairs, good and true, / missed not a step', and at the bottom 'had two stools, / and was translated' out of his senses, to mention just two items from her lengthy confession (5.173–95,124–6). This confession makes Moroso publicly relive his past humiliation. Beyond mocking Moroso at a moment she claims to be admitting guilt and acknowledging her father's authority, Livia targets Moroso's bodily dignity, though not with the same sadistic violence as Petruccio's or Petronius's threats to Maria's body. She, too, thus turns one of the men's tactics of domination against them: Livia takes from Moroso his bodily self-control (and in a way that emphasizes how his old, spent body is unfit for a young bride), just as Petruccio fantasizes he will do to Maria with his cudgels and forced-feeding. Merry-making and eliciting the audience's laughter in response to the claims of Petruccio, Moroso, and their male supporters identify the men's expectations of women as ridiculous. Tricking the men to believe, for a moment, that they really do have authority and that the women really do repent affronting it casts them as foolish dupes for imagining that Maria and Livia, and women in general, will accept their laughable demands.

Eliciting laughter from the audience aligns the laughers with the women's cause, since 'when we laugh we betray our inner-most assumptions'.[102] While laughter might betray inner thoughts as a mind-triggered response, especially in the case of Maria's and Livia's very clever humour, 'Renaissance physicians were primarily interested in laughter as a physical process like breathing or digestion'.[103] They saw laughter as 'an awesome somatic force, sometimes mortally dangerous, sometimes beneficent, capable of breaking through paralysis and clearing

---

[102]   Keith Thomas, qtd in Brown, *Better a Shrew*, 10.
[103]   Brown, *Better a Shrew*, 28.

fistulas'.[104] To incite laughter, then, is to incite a response in audience members that eludes easy definition as mental or corporeal – a response that confuses the hierarchy of intellect or soul over body, the hierarchy that serves as a basic justification for the wife's subjection to the husband.

Even the women's mirthful song and dance combines pleasurable physical abandon – which the audience is invited to join by singing along – with a pointed and clever verbal resonance for the mentally alert. By the time Sophocles tells Petruccio that soon Maria will be under his 'seal', the audience has already witnessed the kind of 'seals' the women enjoy. Indeed, rather than sounding convincing, Sophocles's word choice is a weaker echo of a word the audience has already heard repeated – or perhaps even joined in singing – in the women's lively song of defiance:[105]

> A health, for all this day,
> To the woman that bears the sway,
>> And wears the breeches.
>> Let it come, let it come!
> Let this health be a seal
> For the good of the commonweal
>> The woman shall wear the breeches.
> Let's drink then, and laugh it,
> And merrily, merrily quaff it,
> And tipple and tipple a round.
>> Here's to thy fool
>> And to my fool! (2.5.44–55)

In addition to its definition as a 'device ... impressed on a piece of wax or other plastic material adhering ... to a document as evidence of authenticity or attestation; also, the piece of wax, etc. bearing this impressed device', 'seal' carries a more figurative definition as a 'token or symbol of a covenant; something that authenticates or confirms'.[106] Thus, the phrase 'to set one's seal to' means 'to avouch one's conviction *that*' or 'to express one's assent *to*'.[107] In the women's song, then, toasts of 'wine', 'beer', 'ale', 'cordials', and 'sack' convey their rowdy defiance (2.1.117, 2.5.41, 89, 87), procure their bodily pleasure, and increase their merriment, at the same time marking their serious vow that women will gain ascendancy over men in power relationships – as if their 'seal' is one of the

---

[104] Ibid., 28–9.

[105] In Theatre Erindale's production of the play, the women sang this song repeatedly and it was rather catchy. Brown, *Better a Shrew*, 143–4, reads the song as 'invit[ing] the audience to join in', remarking that 'Ballads often featured a rousing call for participation by customers' and that 'By singing along, as playgoers were known to do, Fletcher's female audiences could take an active role in the pleasurable duty of shaming the men for making violent threats'.

[106] *OED*, 'seal, n.', 2, 1.a and b.

[107] Ibid., 1.c.

ceremonial 'off'rings' Maria refers to earlier.[108] As 'seals', their toasts constitute a token that affirms a vow, symbolically or spiritually, as well as a physical gesture affirming bodily liberty.[109]

As I mention at the outset of this chapter, the techniques I discuss as forming what Fletcher presents as the women's rhetoric are not new tactics, nor are they unique to female characters. Constant reversals of a male opponent's ideas and expectations presented as wonderfully funny also characterize published defences of women such as 'Jane Anger Her Protection for Women' (1589); Rachel Speght's 'A Mouzell for Melastomus' (1617); Ester Sowernam's 'Ester Hath Hang'd Haman' (1617); and Constantia Munda's 'The Worming of a Mad Dogge' (1617). Turning an opponent's arguments against him is not unusual in rhetorical contest. When the debate opens a subject position for women through a female persona, however, such reversals can also reveal how misogynistic and patriarchal arguments justifying the subordination of women to men are really nothing more than arguments – mere rhetorical constructs that can be dismantled and defeated with stronger rhetoric. *The Tamer Tamed* seems to register an awareness that the hierarchical and gendered division between soul and body – which serves as a foundation for the subjection of women to men – is just such a rhetorical construct available for manipulation. And the stronger rhetors in *The Tamer Tamed* are clearly women, with Fletcher tapping into cultural anxiety about the dangers of rhetoric as a tool that played upon the emotions, along with the conventional notion that women were more emotional creatures than were men. Fletcher's play imagines, then, or perhaps bears witness to, a versatile subject position for women that does not invest a sense of self in a positive valuation of the body, or in a construction of body and soul as inseparably merged, but rather in changing forms of opposition to the changing mobilizations of conventional patriarchal structurings of the soul-body hierarchy, which sometimes demarcate and sometimes collapse body and soul in ways oppressive to women. This position, Maria's position, should alert us to the need, then, to place updated considerations of the immaterial alongside the wealth of recent, stimulating study on early modern understandings of the body – to consider the role and meaning of Maria's 'new soul', for instance, and how it defines a struggle that Petruccio mistakenly believes is all about the body.

---

[108] That such alcoholic drinks were also called 'spirits' seems to contribute to their fittingness as yet another means of blurring the conventional divide between soul and body. For a discussion of the alehouse as a 'vitally important site for women's jesting and community life' that questions the critical treatment of 'early modern drinking places' as 'male-dominated milieus that were off limits and off-putting to "respectable" women', see Ch. 2 in Brown's *Better a Shrew*.

[109] Another meaning accrues to the song's 'seal' in that the women sing their song from within a space they have sealed off from men, just as Maria has sealed her body from what she describes as male contamination. In this sense, too, 'seal' contributes to the loosening of the body-spirit distinction, as this physical sealing off seems to preserve the upper chamber as a hallowed space and the female body as 'too divine to handle' (1.3.243).

Chapter 3
Ghost and Haunted

Gender and Stage Ghosts

In *The Lady's Tragedy*, a play of uncertain authorship that most critics now attribute to Middleton,[1] a sustained thematic concern with the soul-body dynamic overlaps with the necessary theatrical interplay between material and immaterial to provide a particularly rich text for examining the tie between soul-body ideas and gender. Performed first in 1611, this early modern play is one of only a few that depict a female ghost. The play foregrounds the soul-body dynamic through the Lady by literally bifurcating her into a soul and a body. The visual juxtaposition of her spirit and corpse resonates with the thematic juxtaposition of the spiritually oriented Lady and the carnally motivated Wife. While considering these layers of engagement with the soul-body relationship, this chapter takes up the interaction between the play's female ghost and the man it haunts as an analogy for that relationship as it was conceptualized in the period, participating in and also pushing against the gender assumptions at its root.

Often, ghosts on the early modern stage, such as Don Andrea in *The Spanish Tragedy* or Hamlet Senior, exercise influence over a character still in the flesh, animating that character and inciting him to action. Other ghosts, such as Susan's in *The Witch of Edmonton* or Banquo's in *Macbeth*, torment the conscience of the haunted so that their mere appearance causes the flesh to tremble.[2] Similarly, the soul's understood position in relation to the body was to animate or give form and motion to the body and to govern the body's urges in accordance with the dictates of reason and morality. The Lady's ghost fulfils the former role in relation to her surviving fiancé and, though more subtly, the latter role as well. The established

---

[1] The play has recently been anthologized as part of *Thomas Middleton: The Collected Works*, ed. Gary Taylor and John Lavagnino. On the case for Middleton's authorship, see Julia Briggs's introduction, 833, to her edition of the play, which appears in Taylor and Lavagnino's *Collected Works*. See also the introduction to Anne Begor Lancashire (ed.), *The Second Maiden's Tragedy*, 19–23. In my use of the title *The Lady's Tragedy* I accept the reasoning Lisa Hopkins, *Female Hero*, 72, offers for this title as opposed to *The Second Maiden's Tragedy*.

[2] While Hamlet famously doubts whether the ghost of his father is an evil spirit sent to mislead him or is his father's soul, reminding us that ghosts and departed souls were not necessarily understood to be the same thing, this doubt does not preclude the possibility that a ghost *could be* the departed soul of a loved one. Hamlet comes to believe he is communicating with his dead father, and in *The Lady's Tragedy* Govianus addresses the Lady's immaterial form as 'ghost', 'spirit', and 'soul', seeming to use these words interchangeably, since he never doubts the apparition's authenticity as the Lady's soul.

genre of body-soul dialogues in English literature, which imagined the soul and body of an individual as distinct personalities arguing with each other, along with the morality play tradition of personifying an individual's abstract qualities, which in some instances involved performatively embodying the soul as a figure separate from the body, gives precedent for reading the Lady's ghost and her fleshly interlocutor as an alternative expression of the soul-body dynamic.[3]

But the portrayal of the Lady's immaterial form as a 'ghost' that haunts its partner adds a new, eerie element to the soul-body dynamic, an eeriness that perhaps bears a similar effect to Gloriana's uncanniness in Middleton's earlier *Revenger's Tragedy* – implying a warning or accusation that the audience can arguably sense but that the haunted does not fully recognize. Ghosts, of course, lack material power to enforce their wishes and must rely on their ability to influence or appeal to the consciences of those who are able to act concretely in the physical world. On some level this position parallels the experience of early modern English women, whose direct participation in public arenas such as politics, law, and formal education beyond childhood was restricted, often leaving them to rely on connections with husbands or other male relations to exercise influence in these spheres. And yet the majority of ghosts that appear on stage were not women, but men. A possible reason that most stage ghosts were 'the revenants of men and of aristocratic men at that', as Ann Jones and Peter Stallybrass explain, is that 'Most stage ghosts have active stakes in inheritance, which is both about the ownership of the future and about the control of memory … They return to claim a future that they "properly" own and that has been taken away from them'.[4] Women were less likely to be perceived as having this 'sense of entitlement and therefore would not have the same claim to sympathy and redress for the loss of property, power, and even life'.[5] In Middleton's tragedy, the Lady's ghost certainly does not seek vengeance for the unjust circumstances of her death, nor does she come to claim an inheritance or a future that was stolen from her or to prevent someone else from assuming her place, even though before the Tyrant's interference she was poised to be a queen, happily betrothed to the rightful king. The Lady's ghost does not even concern herself with restoring to her dethroned fiancé his rightful inheritance as a means of punishing the Tyrant who forced her death. All she wants is to stop the Tyrant from using her corpse as his plaything and to ensure its return to its grave.

---

[3]   Rosalie Osmond, *Mutual Accusation*, discusses the continued popularity of body-soul dialogues into the seventeenth century, as well as the genre's developments from its medieval prototype. See especially Ch. 5. Osmond, 163, also argues that the 'struggle for superiority that is at the heart of the body/soul relationship is intrinsically dramatic, with ultimate salvation or damnation dependent on the outcome'. In Ch. 8, she discusses how 'the relationship thus serves naturally as an analogy to underlie and enrich many other conflicts within the theatre'.

[4]   Ann Rosalind Jones and Peter Stallybrass, *Renaissance Clothing and the Materials of Memory*, 245–68, esp. 261.

[5]   Frances E. Dolan, 'Hermione's Ghost', 224. Dolan is here paraphrasing part of Jones's and Stallybrass's argument.

The only property the Lady lays claim to, in other words, is her own dead body; the only future she strives to control is how that body is interpreted and remembered. In one sense these aims seem humble and private, and highlight her lack of claim to property beyond herself or to the political future of the kingdom. In another sense, however, asserting that her body is her own property *is* a political claim. In the early seventeenth century, ghosts were often associated with the political, frequently appearing in political dreams, for instance, to 'denounce injustices' and 'urge the living to act', as Michelle O'Callaghan observes.[6] Despite the different nature of the Lady's ghost's claims on the living from the usual inheritance-based claims of male ghosts, we can arguably situate the Lady's ghost within this larger tradition of ghosts conveying political meaning, a tradition O'Callaghan sees as stemming from classical ghosts.[7]

Frances Dolan suggests another, more provocative reason for the scarcity of female stage ghosts. Besides reflecting the likelihood that 'dead women were rarely imagined to have legitimate claims on the living', the 'rare appearances of women in ghost stories' might also mean 'that the accusations and demands they might make were too horrifying to imagine'.[8] This chapter seeks to imagine how the seemingly simple demands of the Lady's ghost might in fact get at something deeper and too horrifying for even Govianus to fully recognize. While the ghost might seem to be on a personal errand to restore the sanctity of her grave, this task carries potential to resonate uncomfortably on a political level through its possible comment on gender, a comment that intertwines with the play's treatment of theatricality, as I will explore.

Disembodying Authority in *The Lady's Tragedy*

The Lady's Tragedy features a female character as strong-willed as Maria in *The Tamer Tamed*, who, like Maria, takes charge of her desperate situation and exercises considerable influence over her husband-to-be. Maria's insistence on the connection between her will and her soul, however, inevitably becomes something darker in tragedy: the Lady's firmness of will leads to its violent disembodiment when she literally becomes nothing but soul, a ghost.

The bifurcation of the Lady into spirit and corpse parallels a structural opposition between the virtuous living Lady and her subplot antithesis, the lusty, carnal Wife, in a way that seems to uphold a narrow view of women as either body or soul, either whore or saint. And rather than balancing the negative representation of woman-as-body, the identification of a female character with the soul can have the effect of designating her as exceptional, her strengths as something that real women do not possess on a practical level. Criticism of *The Lady's Tragedy* often

---

6   Michelle O'Callaghan, 'Dreaming the Dead', 81.

7   Ibid., 82.

8   Dolan, 'Hermione's Ghost', 230.

attributes the Lady's formidable resolve, strength, and leadership to her ghostly status as an abstraction of virtue: she is an allegorical figure for Wisdom (drawing on the personification of Wisdom as a woman in Solomon's Book of Wisdom), a figure for spiritual as opposed to carnal orientation, and a figure for the kingdom over which the Tyrant and the true governor struggle.[9]

Although *The Lady's Tragedy* draws on the conventional antithesis between soul and body, setting up a parallel between this antithesis and the misogynistic either/or categorization of women, the play's thematic engagement with soul and body is not static, but shifting and multifaceted. As I will argue in this chapter, the play's fluctuating thematic and performative treatment of the soul-body dynamic often pulls against the limited but common view of women as aligned with either body or soul. The treatment of the soul-body dynamic in *The Lady's Tragedy* further troubles gender assumptions by making gender central to questions the play raises about the difference between tyranny and legitimate authority. To develop this argument I will analyze the play's gendering of the Tyrant along with the Tyrant's associations with the body in juxtaposition with the deposed ruler Govianus, who, though similarly feminized and linked to the body, allows himself to be guided by the Lady's soul. The Lady herself, as soul and even before her death, occupies in relation to Govianus what many in the Renaissance held to be the natural position of the soul in relation to the body – a position of authority and guidance. While the soul was commonly feminized when considered in isolation, this reversal of the predominant gendering of soul and body in relation to each other is uncommon. Through this reversal, *The Lady's Tragedy* presents the Lady as more fit to wield authority than either the legitimate governor or his deposer. The overriding concern of the Lady's ghost, not for Govianus but for her own corpse, prevents her ghost from being contained within an innocuous realm of feminine abstraction, while also suggesting the extent to which the cultural ideal of male governance requires the manipulation of the female body. The Lady's determination to rescue her body from this fate even after death unsettles the distinction between soul and body,

---

9   For the Lady as an allegorical figure of Wisdom alluding to The Wisdom of Solomon, and as a figure for the true kingdom, see Anne Lancashire, *The Second Maiden's Tragedy*, 25, 39. Lancashire, 47, insists that the play does not operate entirely on an allegorical level, but rather presents a 'human drama' instead of 'a piece of abstract moral teaching' (see also 40). The Lady's allegorical significations, however – which Lancashire insightfully identifies and explains – tend to empty the Lady of any potential to challenge male government by acting as a more capable decision maker than any of the play's men, since on some level she serves as 'spiritual guide to good kingship' and 'a symbol of the kingdom's allegiance or love' (42). Sara Eaton, 'Seeing the Emblematic Woman', 68–9, also reads the Lady's body as 'synonymous with the kingdom', a 'territory besieged by the principal male characters'. Focusing on the Lady as 'emblematic woman' leads Eaton to conclude that the Lady's 'final configuration as a sterile and abstracted representation of a queen, a return to an idealized position in Govianus' imagination, is celebrated' (73). Hopkins, *Female Hero*, 44–5, 84–6, reads the play as separating 'actual from symbolic genders' without ever resolving this disjoint that presents '"real" women' negatively.

and thus between the virtuous Lady and her subplot antithesis, the promiscuous Wife. Facing the same misogynistic assumptions discounting their ability to govern even themselves, neither Wife nor Lady can avoid a violent end. Instead of validating the women's fate, *The Lady's Tragedy* stages men facing the destructive repercussions of their own attitudes towards women.

The Lady's Tragedy participates in a long tradition of portraying tyrants and ineffective rulers as effeminate. 'The Platonic tradition', which Rebecca Bushnell identifies as 'primarily responsible for the influential psychological and moral model for tyranny' in the Renaissance, 'describes the tyrant as giving in to excessive desire, which unseats the sovereignty of reason'.[10] Along with the tyrant's irrationality, his 'love of pleasure, his impulse to shift shapes, and his improper sovereignty often generate the accusation that he is, in effect, "feminized"'.[11] Bushnell adds to these stereotypically feminine weaknesses the tyrant's insatiable 'appetite' and his skill at mimesis and deception, or, in other words, his flair for the theatrical.[12] The early modern cultural association between tyranny, effeminacy, and theatricality, which Bushnell traces back to Greek culture, is especially important to a consideration of gender in *The Lady's Tragedy*. 'Attacks on tyranny ... resembled contemporary arguments against the theater', which tended to define theatre as both effeminate and effeminizing.[13] Citing anti-theatrical writings by William Prynne, William Rankins, Stephen Gosson, and Philip Stubbes, Bushnell explains that the actor and the tyrant posed a danger to social and natural order because their outsides did not match their insides; they shifted 'from role to role', failing to display a '"real" or single self on which moral or political character can be grounded'.[14] Problematically, however, legitimate rulers, as both Elizabeth and James demonstrated, acknowledged a need for role-playing in governance, even if they paradoxically constructed their 'princely role' as one of consistency and stability.[15] The use of theatricality that characterizes the typical tyrant, then, also threatens to undermine the distinction between tyrant and legitimate ruler.[16] In *The Lady's Tragedy* a shared theatricality between governor and Tyrant puts into question the very nature of authority and also offers an implicit defence of the theatre, as my analysis will seek to unfold.

---

[10]   Rebecca Bushnell, *Tragedies of Tyrants*, 9–10.

[11]   Ibid., 9.

[12]   Ibid., 20. Bushnell discusses the tyrant's typical effeminacy and theatricality at length, as well as the link between these qualities. See especially 20–25 and 56–69.

[13]   Ibid., 58, 63.

[14]   Ibid., 58–61.

[15]   Ibid., 60. Bushnell notes that 'this need to convey the impression of consistency and integrity when acting a princely role informed both Elizabeth I's and James I's ideology and style of rule. Elizabeth's own motto, *Semper eadem*, privileges consistency, despite her own liberal practice of political theatre. Even more so, James I conceived of himself as "constant as the northern star" yet always on the stage'.

[16]   Ibid., 61.

Anti-theatricalists perceived an even greater danger than deceptive appearances, however, in theatre's stirring of emotion and pleasure. They 'saw plays as inciting both actors and audiences to immoderate desire' at the expense of reason, thus effeminizing all involved.[17]

The Tyrant of *The Lady's Tragedy* certainly exemplifies the connection between tyranny, effeminacy, and theatricality. The Tyrant's excessive desire for the Lady controls his actions. His assumption that the Lady will love whoever is king suggests that his passion is what motivated his seizure of the throne from Govianus, and he determines to abduct and rape the Lady when she refuses him, even though he initially wished for reciprocated affection. If the Tyrant's tenuous grasp on reason was not obvious to his courtiers before, he quickly loses their confidence when, following the Lady's suicide to avoid rape, he steals her corpse from its tomb, fondles it, decorates it in rich clothing and jewels, and has it displayed and attended upon. Anti-theatricalists would find little redeeming value in the effect the Tyrant's actions might have on audience members, who become transfixed voyeurs of his shocking necrophilia, which might be disturbingly erotic, especially if, as Susan Zimmerman points out, an actor played the corpse as opposed to a dummy standing in for it.[18] The Tyrant's theatrical treatment of the Lady's corpse serves as a deceptive display of his own dominance. He employs spectacle to evince that not even death can thwart his will, hiring a disguised Govianus (who is also using theatre to accomplish his own will, here) to 'hide death upon her face' with cosmetic art.[19] The Tyrant's manipulation and presentation of the corpse, dressed to his specifications, is also a show of power over the Lady – who in life denied him her body and even refused to change her attire at his command.[20] As Kevin Crawford claims, the Tyrant's use of the Lady's body additionally signals 'a complete triumph over Govianus's sexual control over her (the Tyrant does possess her, even if she's dead, while Govianus's actions essentially relinquish her to the Tyrant)'.[21] Along with the Tyrant's reliance on theatricality, and especially his turn to cosmetics for help to achieve his unchecked will, his related focus on the body and on materiality fits with the pervasive cultural perception of women as more

---

[17]   Ibid., 62–3. Bushnell points to the way Prynne follows Gosson 'in insisting that plays "effeminate their Actors and Spectators … enervating and resolving the virility and vigor of their mindes, making them mimicall, histrionicall, lascivious, apish, amorous, and unmanly"'. Similarly, anti-theatrical pamphlet writers, as Melinda Gough, 'Jonson's Siren Stage', esp. 69–70, 73–6, points out, repeatedly associate what they deem the dangerously misleading pleasures of the theatre with the charms of a deceptive seductress.

[18]   Susan Zimmerman, *Early Modern Corpse*, 105.

[19]   (5.2.67–9). All citations from *The Lady's Tragedy* refer to Julia Briggs's edition in Taylor and Lavagnino's *Thomas Middleton: The Collected Works*. I cite from the performance version of the text, which appears alongside the original version in this edition.

[20]   Kevin Crawford, 'Softened Masculinity', 105, takes a different view, arguing that the Tyrant's necrophilia 'marks the ultimate softening of his sexual power over the Lady (unsuccessful as conventional masculine wooer, he can have her only in death)'.

[21]   Ibid.

bodily creatures than men.[22] The Tyrant is not the least bit put off, for instance, by the absence of the Lady's spirit, since he values the body above things immaterial, as his identification of the Lady *as* her body and her soul as an inconsequential 'tenant' makes clear (5.2.3).

Perhaps the most significant link, however, among tyranny, effeminacy, and theatricality for my consideration of the play's treatment of women and the soul-body dynamic concerns the idea of usurpation. For John Knox, as Rebecca Bushnell reminds us, any woman who presumes to wield authority over a man is tyrannous, for she does not naturally possess such authority – 'experience hath declared [women] to be inconstant, variable, cruell and lacking the spirit of counsel and regiment'.[23] She thus occupies a position not rightfully hers in claiming authority above a man, just as the Tyrant claims authority that is not rightfully his. Similarly, according to anti-theatrical arguments, theatre promoted a kind of dangerously influential usurpation, with players habitually assuming roles outside their 'natural' gender and station in life. In a sense, both tyrants and women undertaking to govern men were deceptively playing roles that did not belong to them.

The Tyrant's embodiment of stereotypically feminine vices forms part of what Lisa Hopkins identifies as the play's 'distinctly misogynist counter-narrative of femininity', which competes with the positive portrayal of the female protagonist. Hopkins observes this counter-narrative of femininity 'inscribed' in the characters' 'everyday speech', pointing to how Govianus 'strikes the note for the play's sustained demonization of that which is gendered feminine' when he 'excoriat[es] femininity' – by blaming 'False Fortune's sister' for his dethronement – 'even as he deplores the loss of his [beloved Lady]', among other examples.[24] The play indeed perpetuates misogyny through this kind of 'everyday language' along with the Tyrant's implicitly feminine depravities, and even through the framing of Govianus's failure at maintaining proper government as a failure of masculinity.[25] We could also read the Lady's exemplary virtue and actions as owing to her possession of 'masculine' qualities, such as a firm grasp on reason to keep emotions under control, skill with a sword, physical strength, and assertiveness.[26] This alignment of feminine traits with immorality and masculine traits with virtue supports gender hierarchy, even though the immoral character is male and the virtuous hero female. But is the Lady's quickness to sacrifice herself to protect her husband's honour a 'masculine' quality? And

---

[22] For more on associations between theatricality, cosmetics, and women, see Tanya Pollard, *Drugs and Theater*, especially Ch. 4.

[23] John Knox, *First Blast of the Trumpet*, 10; Bushnell, *Tragedies of Tyrants*, 65.

[24] Hopkins, *Female Hero*, 73–7.

[25] Crawford, 'Softened Masculinity', discusses the failed masculinity of all the main male characters as the root of the tragic events.

[26] Ibid., 109, describes the Lady as 'demonstrably more masculine [than Govianus] in confidence and action'.

while the Tyrant's inordinate lust fits with negative views of femininity, is his aggression in pursuing that lust through abduction and planned rape 'feminine'? With the attribution of supposedly feminine traits to the Tyrant and masculine traits to the Lady, cultural distinctions between masculine and feminine become muddied. Even if in one sense affirming gender stereotypes, the Lady's frequent masculinity and the Tyrant's femininity also show that gendered traits are not inherent and are unstable, a possibility that renders gender hierarchy problematic. Similarly, while the play does exemplify conceptual links among the feminine, the tyrannous, and the theatrical, and while, as Crawford suggests, the play even seems to confirm the classical notion that a woman's mere presence could have a disastrous effeminizing effect on men in positions of governmental power,[27] an alternative perspective on tyranny and gender is available alongside – and pushes against – these conceptual links.

Dramatic portrayals of tyrants in the 1610s and 1620s, Bushnell notes, update the morality play characterization of the tyrant as sexually and morally depraved by exploring the relationship between morality and legitimacy, and by focusing on the impact of the tyrant's behaviour on his subjects rather than on his own soul.[28] *The Lady's Tragedy* conveys the Tyrant's destructive impact most fully, however, through a single female subject, the Lady. The men connected to her get off comparatively easy, undergoing fake deaths – Govianus fainting when the Tyrant's henchmen arrive to kidnap the Lady, and her father swooning when Govianus fires a blank pistol to scare him into repentance for serving as the Tyrant's bawd[29] – only the Lady must die for real. The play focuses on the Tyrant's displacement of the Lady's will and usurpation of her body as his main offence – the main expression of his tyranny. This dramatization of illegitimate political authority through the personal oppression of the Lady (and vice versa) troubles the ideal (based on the gender assumptions also in play) of the exclusively male prerogative to govern, both publicly and privately.

The Lady's own ability to govern situations effectively when both men fail to do so supports this potential questioning of the male prerogative to govern. Govianus is the legitimate king and the play constructs an obvious dramatic and moral opposition between him and the usurping Tyrant. Yet from the outset, the Lady's statements and actions direct those around her in pointed contrast to Govianus's uninspiring behaviour – behaviour that Crawford describes as 'weak', 'submissive', and ultimately displaying failed or 'softened' masculinity.[30] When the Tyrant usurps his throne, Govianus indulges publicly in self-pity, blaming 'the adulterate friendship of mankind' for his fall and taking bitter jabs at the defecting nobles, calling them 'ponderous', but only in the sense that their

---

27   Ibid., 101.

28   Bushnell, *Tragedies of Tyrants*, 158.

29   Celia Daileader, *Eroticism on the Renaissance Stage*, 94–5, discusses these male fake deaths as suggesting both sexual and moral failure.

30   Crawford, 'Softened Masculinity', 109–14.

'styles' or titles have become 'heavier', suggesting their acceptance of bribes (1.1.77–9). Govianus assumes that, along with his material possessions, he will lose his betrothed lady, who will inevitably 'snatch her eyes off' him to keep her gaze fixed 'upon advancement', merely because 'she's a woman' (63–7). But while Govianus lumps her with the worldly wealth he must relinquish, the Lady aligns herself with the soul, eternal and unchanging in contrast with the transient body. 'I am not to be altered', she tells the Tyrant in response to his attempts to seduce her with queenship and 'jewels / ... worth ten cities' (101–4). Her subsequent behaviour confirms her declaration, exposing Govianus, in his entire and unwarranted lack of confidence in her, to be as 'ponderous' and fickle as the courtiers he disparages and whom he is supposed to lead.[31] Govianus only regains his kingdom at the end of the play because the Lady's ghost directs him and spurs him to action, animating him the way the soul ideally governs and animates the weaker body, according to inherited Platonic and Aristotelian ideas.

Even in life, the Lady's will and discernment – the highest faculties of the soul according to current English writings on the topic[32] – prove stronger than Govianus's. In his self-absorption the undiscerning Govianus misreads the Lady's first appearance on stage '*clad in black*' (sd after 92). At her entrance he laments, 'Now I see my loss. / I never shall recover't' (92–3). To Govianus's discredit, the Tyrant interprets correctly the Lady's mourning attire as signalling rejection of his triumph. Objecting to her 'widow's case', he commands attendants to 'go, bring me her hither like an illustrious bride' instead (94–103). This is the point at which the Lady declares she is 'not to be altered'. 'I have a mind', she insists, 'that must be shifted ere I cast off these' garments, subordinating her bodily appearance to her inner resolve and refusing to be a vessel for the Tyrant's puppetry. She perceives that her father, however, has become just such a vessel. When he tries to bully her into becoming the Tyrant's mistress, the Lady demands:

> Can you assure me, sir,
> Whether my father spake this, or some spirit
> Of evil-wishing that has, for a time,
> Hired his voice of him to beguile me that way,
> Presuming on his power and my obedience? (2.1.94–8)

In reproaching her father for allowing himself to become a kind of puppet for evil, here, the Lady also indicates that she is not beguiled and that her father's 'power'

---

[31]   Ibid., 110–11, wonders, 'was Govianus a weak, ineffectual ruler who practically asked to be toppled?' Crawford notes that besides blaming false friends instead of 'poor statecraft' for his deposition, and giving up on his betrothed without cause, Govianus lacks 'the strategic wherewithal to accept his sentence of banishment as a boon by which he might return and supplant his ... deposer'. Instead, Govianus resorts to 'whining in a disturbingly Romeo-like fashion' about being separated from the Lady.

[32]   On the will and discernment or understanding as parts of the soul, refer to Ch. 2's section on 'Women, Wit, and Will'.

and her 'obedience' should not be presumed, but depend upon her discernment. In contrast to her father, Govianus, and the Tyrant,[33] the Lady is not 'taken with' 'titles / nor all the bastard honours of this frame' (1.1.106–8). As with Maria in *The Tamer Tamed*, the Lady's resolute will aligns with her soul – that immaterial, unchanging part that governs her outward actions instead of submitting to the temptations of its 'frame', her body. Early modern understandings of the will as 'a natural faculty of the soul' only if it obeys reason, and a 'corruption' and 'infirmity' if it does not, explain the difference between the Lady's insistence on her will and the Tyrant's insistence on his own.[34] The Tyrant exhibits the kind of irrational, wayward wilfulness emerging from physical urges that was stereotypically a female fault. His lustful appetite offsets the Lady's pursuit of her will – as Petruchio's does Maria's in *The Tamer Tamed* – with the effect of presenting female strength of will as a trait to emulate rather than as the proverbial unpredictable force for a man to tame. The Lady's unshakable will sways Govianus in this first scene from pitying himself to deeming himself 'above a king in fortunes' (113).

The enthroned Tyrant even admits, privately, that 'the king walks yonder chose by her affection, / which is the surer side, for where she goes, / her eye removes the court' (127–9), a recognition that perhaps comments on the extent of the Lady's governing influence. The strength of the Lady's will and discernment – which aligns her with the governing soul that she will quite literally become – contrasts most sharply with Govianus's weakness and inaction in the lead-up to her death, a scene in which Govianus confronts, and is paralyzed by, the destructive repercussions of misogyny. The noise of knocking punctuates this suspenseful scene, presumably more violent with each repetition, as the Tyrant's men try to break into Govianus's house. The Lady and Govianus know the men have come to kidnap the Lady for the Tyrant's sexual use. To the Lady's exasperation, the situation immobilizes Govianus: 'have you leisure to stand idle?' she asks, reminding him 'Why, my lord, / It is for *me* they come' (3.1.64–5, emphasis added). This verbal slap in the face calls upon Govianus to look beyond himself and help her. Govianus seems incapable of looking past himself, however, responding in a daze, 'for thee, *my* glory, / the riches of *my* youth, it is for thee' (65–6, emphasis added). The Lady strategizes, envisioning a way to preserve her constant will by separating it, through death, from her body – a body that marks her as a target for the Tyrant's lust. It's a political move, for in addition to saving herself from being 'forced unto' her enemy's 'lust' (95–7), it allows her to protect Govianus, the person she deems the true king. She tells Govianus that she is like 'treasure' sought by 'pirates', 'dangerous to him that

---

[33]   The Lady's father berates her for neglecting the chance to procure 'glory ... for thee and thy seed' and 'advancement for thy father' (2.1.25–6); Govianus initially bemoans the loss of his title and worldly kingdom, counting the Lady among his losses; and the Tyrant believes he can win the Lady with the promise of earthly status and wealth.

[34]   Simon Harward, *Discourse Concerning the Soule*, C4v. See also Ch. 2's section on 'Women, Wit, and Will', which touches upon Renaissance writers who feel the need to explain how the will can be part of the soul and yet capable of committing errors.

keeps it' (70–77). The Lady's sacrifice of her physical body to preserve her soul and will results in the appearance of two bodies onstage – her corpse (either a dummy or an actor) and the actor playing her ghost. These two bodies might loosely recall Queen Elizabeth's rhetoric of the queen's two bodies. To circumvent objections such as that John Knox published during her predecessor's reign, that 'it is more then a monstre in nature, that a woman shall reigne and have empire above man',[35] Elizabeth could appeal to the notion that the monarch was invested with an eternal, unchanging body politic that transcended the infirmities of the flesh, such as age, sickness, and, in her case, gender.[36] Similarly, the Lady seeks to protect her will and to escape a position of weakness framed by her gender: she has no recourse from rape apart from using Govianus's sword as the 'key' which lets her 'slip forth' from her body like a freed 'prisoner' (163). When the Lady urges Govianus to 'dispatch' her (91), however, he cannot face the horrific injustice of her situation:

> O, this extremity!
> Hast thou no way to 'scape 'em, but in soul?
> Must I meet peace in thy destruction,
> Or will it ne'er come at me?
> 'Tis a most miserable way to get it. (82–5)

Physically trapped with the Lady in the room under siege, Govianus also comes up against the cultural trap she faces. As the Lady puts it, the Tyrant's 'lust may part thee from me, but death, never' (144), for once the Tyrant destroys her honour, Govianus could never 'enjoy' her but would rather 'curse / that love that sent forth pity to [her] life' (146, 79–80). The tendency to define women as either saints or whores depending on their sexual status leads to this 'extremity' that Govianus balks at – the Lady can ''scape in soul' or be forever ruined in body (82).

The Lady frames Govianus's inability to help her achieve her will as a failure to govern the situation. After urging him to act like 'a resolute captain' and one who is 'master yet' of his house, she berates him for letting her face the Tyrant's injustice alone:

> Sir, you do nothing. There's no valour in you.
> You're the worst friend to a lady in affliction
> That ever love made his companion!
> For honour's sake, dispatch me! Thy own thoughts
> Should stir thee to this act more than my weakness.
> The sufferer should not do't. I speak thy part,
> Dull and forgetful man, and all to help thee! (88–94)

---

[35] Knox, *First Blast of the Trumpet*, A3v–A4.

[36] For discussion of Elizabeth's strategic use of the notion of the monarch's two bodies, see Marie Axton, *The Queen's Two Bodies*; Theodora A. Jankowski, *Women in Power*, 60–62. Eaton, 'Seeing the Emblematic Woman', 80, also suggests that the Lady's 'doubleness' embodies 'for the audience the familiar contemporary understandings of the Queen's two bodies'.

The Lady must do more than speak Govianus's part, however, for when he finally musters the nerve to run at her with a sword, he '*falls by the way in a swoon*' (149 sd), leaving the Lady to reflect:

> O thou poor-spirited man!
> … Did I trust to thee,
> And hast thou served me so? Left all the work
> Upon my hand, and stole away so smoothly?
> There was not equal suffering shown in this. (150–54)

As much as the Lady stands as an allegorical figure for wisdom or for the way of the spirit, she is very human here in her disappointment in the man to whom she has pledged herself. And even though her quest for death is hardly liberating, these passages are stirring with almost proto-feminist sentiment in their recognition that the Lady is the real 'sufferer' and that even though he is not in her position – in fact *because* he is not in her position – Govianus has a responsibility to act, to acknowledge and face the injustice alongside her, and to honour her will. Abandoned in her time of need, however, the Lady is not at a loss. Addressing Govianus's sword as she takes it up, she claims,

> … thou hast lost
> A fearful master, but art now preferred
> Unto the service of a resolute lady,
> One that knows how to employ thee, and scorns death
> As much as some men fear it. (157–60)

The sword is a phallic symbol of male power and authority linked to the sceptre that the Lady rejects from the Tyrant in the opening scene,[37] adding weight to the Lady's assertion that she knows how to use it.

The Wife, the Lady's subplot antithesis, is another woman who knows how to use, and dies by, a sword. Whereas the Lady tries to escape 'in soul' an unjust situation, the Wife attempts to escape an unfair situation in body, which makes her the whore to the Lady's saint. Just as, prior to meeting the Lady, we witness Govianus wrongfully speaking ill of her, before we meet the Wife we see her husband, Anselmus, needlessly obsessing about her chastity. Unable to trust her self-government, Anselmus decides that a wife who is 'thought good' is not enough. His wife must be 'approved so' (1.2.36) by resisting his friend Votarius's attempts to seduce her. A shocked Votarius tries to dissuade Anselmus, asking, 'must a man needs, in having a rich diamond, / put it between a hammer and an anvil / and … / break it in pieces to find out the goodness' (53–6)? This early warning places the blame for what will unfold entirely on Anselmus. Before setting his wife between a hammer and an anvil, however, Anselmus makes her fragile. Seeking Anselmus but finding Votarius instead (Anselmus is hiding to spy on her), the Wife confides:

---

[37]   Crawford, 'Softened Masculinity', 102–3, notes the link between sceptre and sword as phallic symbols in the play.

> I want [Anselmus's] company.
> He walks at midnight in thick shady woods
> ...
> ... I have watched him
> ...
> Stood in my window, cold and thinly clad,
> T'observe him ...
> ...
> And when the morning dew began to fall,
> Then was my time to weep. He's lost his kindness,
> Forgot the way of wedlock, and become
> A stranger to the joys and rites of love.
> He's not so good as a lord ought to be.
> Pray, tell him so from me, sir. (98–111)

The Wife, like the Lady, turns to a man for help, although in a different kind of desperation: she is desolate, emotionally and physically neglected by her husband, because, as we know, he is busy fretting about how to test her. And while Govianus simply proves useless in the Lady's hour of need, the man to whom the Wife turns actively seduces her instead of being her advocate with Anselmus. While criticism on *The Lady's Tragedy* habitually discusses the Lady and the Wife as morally instructive opposites, then, with one making all the right choices and the other confirming all the worst stereotypes about women,[38] we gain an entirely different perspective by focusing on the men that drive the Lady and the Wife to their opposite 'extremities'.

A difference in sensory perception highlights the difference in personality between the brothers, Anselmus and Govianus. Anselmus is preoccupied with sight: he seeks visual proof of the Wife's chastity and wants to watch as Votarius tempts her. Govianus, by contrast, is not sight-oriented, as his failure to even notice the Lady's mourning garments that so upset the Tyrant makes clear. Govianus instead responds to sound. The Lady's words, not her appearance, transform him in the first scene, and before the Lady's ghost appears to Govianus in the tomb she penetrates his thoughts as a disembodied voice, claiming, 'I am not here' (4.4.40). When the ghost does emerge, she emphasizes, 'I come to *tell* you all my wrongs' (54, emphasis added). The significance of this difference lies in the early modern understanding of sight as projective (eyes shot beams out at objects to perceive them) and hearing as receptive (the ear received sound as a 'feminized perceptual organ').[39] Our current 'predominantly visual culture', as Wes Folkerth claims, 'has

---

[38] See, for example, Hopkins, *Female Hero*, 72–3, 81, 86; Richard Levin, 'The Double Plot of *The Second Maiden's Tragedy*', 219–31; Lancashire, *The Second Maiden's Tragedy*, 34.

[39] By the end of the sixteenth century, as Eric Langley, 'Anatomizing the Early-Modern Eye', explains, two competing perceptions of the eye existed. While the new scientific understanding of the eye as a receptive and fragile organ came to replace the Platonic and Galenic models of the active eye projecting eyebeams in order to see, the older, projective

come to privilege' 'values of mastery, dominance, and invulnerability', while early modern people associated hearing with 'duty', 'receptivity', 'transformation', and 'community'.[40] Anselmus's fixation on sight thus codes his approach to his wife as aggressive and his negative view of her as essentially coming from within himself and pushed onto her. Govianus, however, lets the Lady's words change his idea of her and of wealth early on, and continuing to listen to her eventually leads him back to the throne. His receptive nature perhaps explains the Lady's loyalty to him (we can't really credit his resolute will or leadership skills), while Anselmus's aggressiveness and self-centredness lead the Wife and Votarius to deceive him through appearances. When this deception comes to light, Anselmus ends up flinging the Wife's corpse away from him in disgust, calling her 'a whore' and vowing that he would rather 'sup with torments' in hell than see her in heaven (5.1.170–77). This invective comes mere moments after Anselmus has declared himself happy to die 'close by the chaste side of my virtuous mistress' (11). Anselmus's extreme views of women as either pure or evil lead him to these violent emotional extremes. And yet, whereas Govianus comes to understand, but cannot face, the Lady's predicament, Anselmus, in flinging the Wife's corpse from him, refuses to recognize how his views have destroyed the Wife and himself.[41]

Even though the Lady took drastic measures to avoid the Wife's fate of being judged a whore, the Tyrant violates her body after death. The Lady's ghost wants to rescue her body from the Tyrant, who, she relates, 'folds me within his arms and often sets / a sinful kiss upon my senseless lip' (4.4.71–2). 'My rest is lost', she tells Govianus, 'thou must restore't again' (79). The ghost's concern for her body asserts a connection between spirit and flesh that problematizes the dichotomous thinking separating the Lady from the Wife. Her language aligns subjectivity with her corpse and with her soul by assigning first-person personal pronouns to each: she claims 'I am not here' (in body), and yet 'I come to tell you all my wrongs' (in spirit). Performance would emphasize this inseparability of soul and body, the lack of distance between saintly lady and sinful wife. Not only does performance use physical means to shape an audience's ideas about ghostliness – from movement to costume fabrics and makeup – but the stage directions indicate that the ghost appears in the same clothing and jewellery as her body does after the Tyrant has dressed the corpse in a new robe. Moreover, Richard Robinson, the actor who played the living Lady, also played her ghost and, as Lancashire explains, he could

---

model of the eye with its eyebeams, while increasingly out of favour scientifically, remained a recognized metaphor in poetic heritage, and continued to circulate in literature. Langley discusses how both the eyebeams of 'poetic heritage' and the latest scientific model of the receptive eye are both at work in Phineas Fletcher's 1633 *The Purple Island*. I'd like to thank Mary Silcox for pointing me to useful sources on Renaissance theories of vision. On the ear as receptive organ see Wes Folkerth, *Sound of Shakespeare*, 10.

[40]   Folkerth, *Sound of Shakespeare*, 9–10.

[41]   Lancashire, *The Second Maiden's Tragedy*, 45, also observes that the play invites us to blame Anselmus, though Anselmus does not recognize his fault.

have easily doubled as the Wife.[42] What might it mean, then, that the Lady's ghost returns to remove her corpse from the Tyrant's use, apart from the belief that the body's proper burial was necessary for the soul's repose and eventual reunion with the body on the last day?[43] The Wife's escape in body from her emotional turmoil would be seen as detrimental to her soul, but the Lady's escape in soul ends up being detrimental to her body, leaving it for the Tyrant's manipulation after all, and even to Govianus's, for just as the men measured their power in relation to each other by the living Lady's allegiance, they continue to demonstrate their authority through displaying the Lady's corpse.[44]

The Tyrant, like Vindice in *The Revenger's Tragedy*, manipulates the body of the woman he professed to love, making it conform to his own plans and desires. As with Vindice, assuming control over the female body in this way amounts to assuming control over death, and this conflation similarly highlights the arrogance of subordinating the female body to male displays of power. The Tyrant imposes on the Lady's corpse the position and the symbols she refused in life, ornamenting it with rich jewels, having it carried to him in a chair, and instructing his soldiers to '*make obeisance to her*' as if she were now enthroned his queen, publicly supporting his reign instead of standing by the deposed Govianus and symbolically maintaining his kingship through her 'affection' (5.2.sd after 15, 1.1.123–7). As Zimmerman phrases it, the Tyrant 'retaliates' against the Lady's resistance 'by establishing, through violent means, a fetishistic surrogate for the Lady's living body over which he has absolute power'.[45] Insisting that his 'pleasure shall prevail' despite the Lady's rejection and subsequent death, the Tyrant determines to 'force beauty on yon lady's face' through 'art', and to 'labour life into her' with his 'arms and lips' (5.2.96–8, 104–5). He reveals, here, both a delusional confidence in his ability to somehow animate the corpse with the intensity of his desire[46] and a reliance on artifice to achieve and demonstrate possession of Govianus's last treasure. He turns to theatrical artifice in particular, with the adornment and

---

[42] Lancashire, *The Second Maiden's Tragedy*, 54–5. See also Daileader, *Eroticism on the Renaissance Stage*, 94, and for further discussion about how staging blurs the line between the Lady's corpse and spirit, see Zimmerman, *Early Modern Corpse*, 104.

[43] The Lady and Govianus both allude to this belief. See 3.1.134–7 and 5.2.137. In the first passage, the Lady compares her soul's imminent departure from her body to one 'removing from her house' who has locked up all her goods for safekeeping (her goods represent her words, according to the logic of the comparison) and does not wish to disturb them during the brief time she remains in her house before leaving, so makes do with anything else available. The idea of locking up goods for safekeeping implies an eventual return to the house. In the second passage, Govianus assures the Lady that her 'body shall return [to its grave] to rise again'.

[44] Eaton, 'Seeing the Emblematic Woman', 69, similarly claims that 'the Tyrant and Govianus define their sense of political worth sexually, in terms of the idealized possession of the Lady'.

[45] Zimmerman, *Early Modern Corpse*, 101.

[46] Ibid., 102, makes this point.

procession of the corpse and gestures of homage towards it, and with his call for cosmetics 'To give our eye delight in that pale part' (5.2.99–101). The Tyrant defines and displays his position of power through his possession and control of this female body.

Govianus, too, uses the Lady's corpse in a theatrical way to make his own statement, which troubles the distinctions between what Govianus and the Tyrant ostensibly stand for: legitimate authority versus tyranny based on usurpation, morality versus corruption.[47] Also like *The Revenger's Tragedy*'s Vindice, Govianus exacts revenge upon his enemy by painting the Lady's face and lips with poisonous cosmetics to entice the Tyrant into a fatal kiss. Govianus thus casts the Lady in the role of seductive and deceptive prostitute – the role that she, like Gloriana, killed herself in order to avoid. While Govianus can claim that he is acting on his deceased lady's behalf with more credibility than Vindice can, since we witness the Lady's ghost spurring Govianus to remove her body from the Tyrant's clutches, murdering the Tyrant is, of course, in his own best interest – it clears the throne that is rightfully his. And when Govianus finds himself heartily welcomed back to that throne, he employs the Lady's corpse as the first image of his new reign, crowned, enthroned, and carried offstage[48] in solemn procession to music – an image that recalls the Tyrant directing her earlier procession onstage in a chair and also to music.

Like the Tyrant, Govianus uses the Lady's body to legitimize his reign and to present a desired image of himself – perhaps as his Lady's avenger and as the king whom the Lady herself chose when she was alive. Such a reminder would provide a much needed boost to Govianus's masculinity in the eyes of the court in that, as Crawford notes with reference to Elizabeth Foyster's work on early modern manhood, male sexual dominance was evident not through physical coercion of a woman, but through the ease with which a man persuades a woman to freely choose him.[49] The Tyrant's resort to rape and necrophilia constitutes the

---

[47]   Several critics point out moments when differences between Govianus and the Tyrant collapse. See, for instance, Bushnell, *Tragedies of Tyrants*, 154–6; Crawford, 'Softened Masculinity', 113–14; Zimmerman, *Early Modern Corpse*, 99; Pollard, *Drugs and Theater*, 103–4.

[48]   Govianus speaks lines narrating the Lady's crowning and enthronement in the original version ('here place her in this throne, crown her our queen, / The first and last that ever we make ours, / Her constancy strikes so much firmness in us' [5.2.201–3]), but these lines were cut from the performance version. The removal of these lines, however, does not for certain indicate that the body was *not* enthroned and crowned before it was carried offstage – indeed, silence might add more gravity to these symbolic gestures. The lines immediately preceding the cut lines remain in the record of the performed version: ''tis our will / it [the Lady's body] receive honour dead, as it took part / With us in all afflictions when it lived' (5.2.154–6). These remaining lines leave room for such a crowning to take place before the Lady's spirit appears '*and stays to go out with the body, as it were attending it*' (sd after 156).

[49]   Crawford, 'Softened Masculinity', 104.

'ultimate softening of *his* sexual power over the Lady', then, while also serving to compensate by bringing a sense of absolute control over a body that can no longer argue or resist.[50] Literary critics have described in different ways how both the Tyrant and Govianus define their respective political and social positions in terms of their relationship to the Lady.[51] This conflation of their political and social power with their command of the Lady's loyalty speaks to the ideological connection between a husband's authority within marriage and a king's authority within his kingdom. Both the Tyrant and Govianus feel that their hold on the affection of the Lady, whom they both desire as a wife, corresponds to their hold on the kingdom. When the Lady first refuses the newly crowned Tyrant's love, for instance, he questions whether he has indeed just won the throne:

> Sure some dream crowned me.
> If it were possible to be less than nothing,
> I wake, the man you seek for. There's the kingdom
> Within yon valley [i.e., Govianus] fixed, while I stand here
> Kissing false hopes upon a frozen mountain,
> Without the confines. (1.1.121–6)

As discussed earlier in this chapter, Govianus, on the flip side, is absolutely convinced that because he has lost the kingdom to the Tyrant he has also lost the Lady to him – until the Lady persuades them both otherwise. For both men, male authority and female compliance are interdependent or mutually defining, such that Govianus cannot imagine the Lady remaining faithful to him once he has failed publicly at demonstrating his male authority, and the Tyrant cannot fathom the Lady refusing him once he has become the male authority governing the kingdom. This reliance on female submission to make visible or justify male authority degenerates into both men literally manipulating the Lady's lifeless corpse to reassert their ability to govern.

These similarities between the Tyrant and the rightful ruler make it difficult to distinguish legitimate authority from usurped and abused power. The Lady's superior demonstration of assertiveness and leadership further troubles the legitimacy of male authority as something defined against female submission, especially given the play's historical context of nostalgia for a martial, active Queen Elizabeth, and the critical climate surrounding the pacifist King James.[52]

---

[50]   Ibid., 105–6.

[51]   See, for instance, n. 44; Crawford, 'Softened Masculinity', 102; and Lancashire, *The Second Maiden's Tragedy*, 39, 42, who describes the Lady as symbolic of the kingdom over which the Tyrant and Govianus struggle.

[52]   The turn towards nostalgia for Queen Elizabeth and increasingly critical perspectives on James have been well studied. See, for instance, Eaton, 'Seeing the Emblematic Woman', 80–81, citing John N. King and Roy Strong: 'King suggests that "Jacobean politics provided a motive for the anachronistic revival of the cult of Elizabeth as a model ruler whose perpetual virginity symbolized political integrity, Protestant ideology, and a militantly

The Lady's decisiveness under pressure and her ability to act aggressively, slaying herself with a sword in order to prevent the Tyrant's victory and rape, aligns her with contemporary romanticized concepts of Elizabeth as an extremely effective female ruler, while Govianus's comparative passivity and the need to repeatedly spur him to action align him with negative perceptions of James's pacifism as a failure to advance the Protestant cause. The play, as Lancashire cautions, does not function as a sustained political allegory.[53] These evocations of the current king and the previous queen, however, combine with the Lady's associations with the animating soul and Govianus's with the serving body in a way that exerts pressure on the ideal – perhaps most vehemently articulated by Knox – of governing authority as a distinctly male prerogative and trait, both in individual relationships and in a wider political arena.

At the same time, Govianus's final appropriation of the Lady's image during the process of offstaging her body bears resemblance to James's use of Elizabeth's still powerful image paired with his relocation of Elizabeth's body to a less central tomb. 'When Govianus explains his plan to crown the corpse queen before reburying it', Melissa Walters claims, 'he fully exposes the function of the chaste lady as legitimizer of governmental authority'.[54] The Lady's chastity, in other words, functions as a sign of honour and submission to Govianus as her lord, rather than as a demonstration of her personal integrity. For Sheetal Lodhia, 'now that the "contest of masculinity" [between Tyrant and king] is over', Govianus's crowning of the corpse 'marks his triumph materially'.[55] Sara Eaton finds that this use of the Lady's body depends upon a kind of erasure of the Lady herself so that 'her final configuration', enthroned and carried away at the play's end, is 'as a sterile and abstracted representation of a queen'. Instead of sharing in Govianus's power, the only victory that seems to await her is to occupy 'an idealized position in Govianus' imagination'; 'the Lady's voice' ultimately 'dies with her'.[56] Govianus's self-serving use of the Lady's image might recall King James's use of Elizabeth's image in that 'Shortly before [*The Lady's Tragedy* was] produced, both Mary Stuart's and Elizabeth's elaborate Monumental tombs had been completed, helping James to "construct a political legitimacy with a continuous history"'.[57] 'James's need for visualized "legitimacy" coincided with

---

interventionist policy against Spain. Because these values were increasingly found wanting at the court of England's Scottish king, Protestant militants praised the late queen in order to attack Jacobean pacifism." As Roy Strong has noted, Elizabeth's portraits and impresas enjoyed widespread continued popularity because they exposed a gap between the "poetic dream of the peace and justice of the empire embodied in the state portraits of the Queen and the grim realities of the political scene"'. See also Carole Levin, *'Heart and Stomach of a King'*, 168–9, and Kevin Sharpe, *Selling the Tudor Monarchy*, 467, 473.

[53]   Lancashire, *The Second Maiden's Tragedy*, 38–40, 44.

[54]   Melissa Walter, 'Dramatic Bodies and Novellesque Spaces', 75–6.

[55]   Sheetal Lodhia, 'Material Self-Fashioning and Revenge Tragedy', 145.

[56]   Eaton, 'Seeing the Emblematic Woman', 72–3.

[57]   Ibid., 80.

and', as Eaton suggests, 'perhaps created the conditions for what John N. King terms [the] "sentimental idealization of the late queen", which can be documented in plays, masques, and histories'.[58] But besides completing these statement monuments, James also transferred Elizabeth's tomb to 'the marginal space of the north aisle' from its previous position 'under the altar of the Henry VII Chapel in Westminster Abbey', a 'place of priority' that James reserved for himself.[59] Govianus thus echoes James's approach to his predecessor by finally casting the Lady in a supporting role: rather than acknowledging his debt to her leadership and direction, he gives 'reverence' to her 'chastity' and honours her 'body', not for its own trials but because 'it took part / with us in all afflictions when it lived' (5.2.152–6). The Lady's virtuous image is useful to Govianus, as Elizabeth's was to James, but ultimately he, too, conjures that image in order to displace it. In light of the contemporary nostalgia for Elizabeth as the more effective ruler, these potential evocations of James through Govianus might encourage a critical view of Govianus. Or, they might simply reflect a cultural norm or expectation of male precedence over women in official positions of government.

The similarities between the Tyrant and Govianus in their willingness to use the Lady's corpse for their own purposes, however, should not completely obscure the significant differences in their perceptions of the Lady's body. While both men turn the corpse into a theatrical spectacle, literalizing, in effect, the existing anti-theatrical and misogynistic associations between theatre and femininity reviewed earlier in this chapter, their respective approaches to this spectacle suggest very different understandings of theatre. The Tyrant turns the Lady's body into an idol, as Zimmerman discusses at length, and his privileging of the material over the spiritual corresponds with a gross over-valuing of the self, manifest in the Tyrant's conviction that he himself can animate the corpse through 'his own erotic energy' and 'an act of his will'.[60] His hostility towards the Lady's spirit when it appears to him suggests his rejection of any abstract meaning the corpse might possess beyond the material pleasure it affords him. Tanya Pollard describes the Tyrant as consuming and merging with the spectacle he gazes on, confusing the boundary 'between watching, directing, and participating' in theatrical spectacle with 'toxic consequences'.[61] The notion of theatre as something to be consumed fits with the anti-theatrical contentions that theatre incites inordinate lust and fosters idle pleasure-seeking. For Pollard, the Tyrant's fatal inability to separate himself from spectacle warns about the potential dangers of theatre as addictive, seductive, and deceptive.[62]

---

[58] Ibid.

[59] Julia M. Walker, 'Bones of Contention', 252–4. Levin, *'Heart and Stomach of a King'*, 168, notes that James built Elizabeth 'a magnificent monument', but that 'most of the ceremonial that spring was welcoming James rather than mourning Elizabeth'.

[60] See Zimmerman, *Early Modern Corpse*, 96–106.

[61] Pollard, *Drugs and Theater*, 102–5.

[62] Ibid., Ch. 4.

But this warning is not the only meta-fictional perspective on theatricality that the play offers. I have highlighted the troubling similarity between Govianus and the Tyrant in their theatrical treatments of the corpse, but this similarity – which does indeed undermine the ostensible moral opposition between tyrant and legitimate ruler in a productive way for a study of gender in the play – is limited. Govianus essentially pits one understanding of theatricality against another: he employs theatricality, in the form of the painted corpse, to counter and correct the Tyrant's abuse of theatricality and misinterpretation of materiality. Unlike the Tyrant, Govianus is not guilty of idolatry: he does not value the corpse in and of itself, but for its connection to the Lady's soul. He follows that soul's direction and demonstrates an acute awareness of the body's continuing importance for the soul. Far from being taken with the painted corpse, Govianus is fully aware of the illusion he is creating and even hesitates to present the material body in a way that is incongruous with its soul, its deeper meaning, claiming,

> A religious trembling shakes me by the hand
> And bids me put by such unhallowed business,
> But revenge calls for't, and it must go forward.
> 'Tis time the spirit of my love took rest.
> Poor soul, 'tis weary, much abused and toiled. (5.2.77–81)

And when he indulges in a display of the Lady's corpse that helps legitimize his return to kingship in the final scene, the appearance of the Lady's ghost to escort her body back to its grave prompts Govianus to defend himself, perhaps betraying a sense of guilt at exploiting her body for self-promoting purposes: he assures the spirit, 'thou need'st not mistrust me' (158).[63] Govianus recognizes that the corpse is dead but, because of the spirit that once inhabited it, not empty of meaning – it will 'rise again' to reunite with the soul on the last day, and in the meantime, its desecration torments the Lady's soul (137). The Tyrant is content to forget the former 'tenant' of the Lady's body and, like Vindice in *The Revenger's Tragedy*, impose his own meaning on the Lady's corpse, casting it in a role the Lady refused while living. Govianus refuses to see the Lady's corpse as anything other than her corpse – he does not over-invest in the material, yet he acknowledges a responsibility towards it, a need to ensure it is not mishandled and misinterpreted, for the sake of the Lady's spirit, the something deeper it remains somehow connected to if not animated by.

The contrast between Govianus's balanced, practical, and respectful approach to the Lady's corpse, and the Tyrant's delusional and disturbing infatuation with it, arguably presents two possible understandings of theatre's materiality, especially since the play engages overtly with the politics of theatrical display through the dressing, adorning, and painting of the Lady's corpse at the culmination of the Tyrant's and Govianus's struggle for power. In his deluded belief that the

---

[63]   Lodhia, 'Material Self-Fashioning and Revenge Tragedy', 145, emphasizes Govianus's defensiveness here, and suggests that the Lady's presence signals her distrust.

cosmeticized corpse is on the verge of coming to life, the Tyrant falls into the kind of trap that anti-theatricalists warned theatre sets for spectators – he over-values the material and is seduced and fooled by false appearances. The Tyrant's resort to necrophilia and his unabated infatuation for the Lady's dead body is so extreme, however, that rather than serving as a cautionary tale, he entertains with the shock value of his excessive behaviour, like his medieval cycle play predecessor, Herod. Everyone recognizes and no one shares his insane and skewed perspective – not even his soldiers can refrain from expressing their horror at the Tyrant's simultaneous lack of respect for the material body and his unnatural obsession with it when he robs the Lady's grave. The soldiers and Govianus exemplify the normal perception of the corpse as something that, paradoxically, does not merit adoration or affection in and of itself, and yet does contain value for what it signifies beyond itself – the Lady and her sacrifice. The juxtaposition of Govianus's and the Tyrant's relationships to the Lady's body works to defend the value of theatrical materiality in that only someone as delusional and self-absorbed as the Tyrant could indulge in such a gross misreading and misuse of the material. Even more significantly, though, in Govianus's hands theatre becomes an instrument to defeat corruption and restore political order in the kingdom.

The Lady's ghost's own determination to rescue her material body from the Tyrant's abuse and wrongful interpretation supports this implicit defence of theatre, an art which, of necessity, relies on materiality. Like her corpse, theatre's materiality can be misinterpreted as fostering empty idolatry and obscuring spiritual truths when it really conveys meaning that reaches beyond the material, just as the corpse is connected to the Lady's spirit.[64] And in this play, as in *The Revenger's Tragedy* and *Bartholomew Fair*, the assertion of value in the material and the blurred line between matter and spirit are inextricable from a comment on gender relations in women's favour. *The Lady's Tragedy* goes much further with this comment than the other plays, though, by portraying a female character who, when literally divided into the two components of flesh and spirit, expresses – as a ghost – active and relentless concern for her body. As in the other plays I have so far discussed, this claim for the body's worth and for its continual connectedness to the soul exists alongside and pushes against another current of thought that devalues the body as the antithesis of the soul: unruly, lustful, and vulnerable to corruption. The violent split between the Lady's spirit and body links thematically with the main expression of this negative view of the body: the dramatic opposition between the virtuous, spiritually oriented Lady and the carnally motivated Wife,

---

[64] This assertion that valuing the body does not amount to idolatry might seem an oddly Catholic sentiment coming from a playwright noted for his Protestant leanings (if Middleton is indeed responsible for *The Lady's Tragedy*), but it is unsurprising if we keep in mind that, as Ch. 1 discusses, anti-Catholicism and anti-theatricalism overlapped in objections to elaborate material display. A validation of theatre's value that accounts for its material medium cannot avoid seeming a little 'Catholic' in refusing to entirely denounce spectacle or to maintain a rigid line between body and soul.

especially since the Tyrant, through dressing up, bejewelling, and painting the Lady's corpse, essentially turns it into the figure of a whore – the opposite of the chaste spirit that formerly inhabited it. This strong thematic connection is relevant to the question I posed earlier in this chapter about what the Lady's determination to rescue her body might mean. The ghost's concern for her abused and misrepresented body asserts an enduring, even death-defying link between soul and body which implicitly criticizes the cultural tendency to polarize women as either spiritual or bodily, perfectly virtuous or irredeemably sinful. On some level, then, the ghost's return for her body also rescues or reinterprets the Wife's thrown-away corpse. In reclaiming her own body from the wrongful signification imposed by the Tyrant, the ghost casts a critical light on the signification Anselmus imposes on the Wife's body when he flings it away from him as though he has nothing to do with her ruin. Indeed, just as the Tyrant fashions the corpse into the image of a whore, Anselmus's preconceived conviction of the Wife's infidelity and his resulting unnatural behaviour towards her are what essentially turn the Wife into the figure of a whore. Given the above-mentioned likelihood that the same actor played both the Lady and the Wife, performance would lend support to this reading of the ghost's concern for her abused corporal counterpart as holding meaning that also resonates in the subplot.

The ghost's desire to remove her body from the Tyrant also resonates with the questions the play raises about legitimate authority and government and their relationship to gender. As this chapter has explored, male characters – legitimate and illegitimate rulers alike – perceive their control over the female body as a marker of their authority. Even Govianus, in the first scene, sees the Lady as a trophy he has lost in a contest of male power. The Lady reveals her awareness that the Tyrant is not the only one responsible for her fate the moment she reminds Govianus that if she does not die to escape the Tyrant's rape, she will still be lost to Govianus, who would thereafter never be able to 'enjoy' her. Govianus's immediate acceptance of this logic affirms that the Lady cannot occupy a middle ground – that another man's manipulation of her body can determine her worth, changing her from pure to tainted, saint to whore. This view – which the Lady herself seems to share – traps the Lady within her body, a body that also makes her a target for the Tyrant's lust and a liability to Govianus. Her body is also what bars her from officially exercising the kind of governing authority that the Tyrant seizes and that Govianus regains, despite the fact that her actions reveal her to be far more suited than either man for such a position. Both men subject the Lady to a tyranny of the body (and Anselmus does the same to the Wife). Their treatment of her as an object to be claimed or lost disregards her soul as the rightful 'governor' and decision maker for her body – the issue of her consent does not end up mattering to either the Tyrant or Govianus. The fact that control over the Lady's body continues to define the power struggle between the Tyrant and Govianus after her spirit has vacated that body underlines this point. The very presence of the ghost challenges the usurpation of authority over her body and calls upon Govianus to take responsibility for its abuse in much the same way that the Lady urged him (unsuccessfully) to take responsibility for her predicament when the Tyrant's henchmen arrived to abduct her. Indeed, beyond signalling her trust in him, the Lady's demands for Govianus to help could equally suggest that she views him as complicit in her entrapments.

The actor's gestures, facial expressions, and tone would be essential indicators of the ghost's mood and attitude towards Govianus, but without knowing these details, we can allow for the possibility of the ghost appearing annoyed, angry, even accusatory towards him. She always addresses Govianus honourably as 'dear lord' or 'true lord', and affectionately as 'my truest love' when he informs her that the Tyrant is dying and 'has no power / to vex thee further' (4.4.54, 80, 5.2.136–9), and yet the ghost's abrupt speeches, juxtaposed with Govianus's flowery praise for the Lady at her tomb, imply her impatience with him. Perhaps not coincidentally, the ghost first chooses to appear soon after Govianus, commending his page for the performance of a sorrowful song, tells the boy 'thy better years shall find me good to thee / when understanding ripens in thy soul, / which truly makes the man' (4.4.32–4). This timing of her first appearance makes a silent but critical addition to Govianus's gender-exclusive words, since the sight of the Lady's disembodied soul sharply recalls her willingness to sacrifice her body for her soul – something Govianus could not overcome the weakness of his own body to do. The ghost's initial words interrupt Govianus's apostrophe to the Lady's body with a curt 'I am not here', and her entrance, '*on a sudden in a kind of noise like a wind*' with '*doors clattering*' and the tombstone flying open (sd following 41), certainly does not evince an effort to put Govianus at ease. He expresses 'delight' mingled with 'terror' and 'astonishment' at the apparition of his loved one – the expected reaction to seeing a ghost and yet one that could also suggest a latent sense of guilt towards the Lady – the guilt that again surfaces at the ghost's final appearance to see her corpse back to its resting place. The legacy of literary ghosts appearing in political dreams or materializing onstage to reclaim lost property or a damaged reputation adds impact to the Lady's seemingly simple quest to restore the sanctity of her grave. Essentially, she is making a political statement by asserting ownership over her body and control over the meaning of her death as an act that demonstrated that ownership through refusing the male treatment of her body as a marker of their own political authority, the 'treasure' of their power struggle. Paradoxically, given that a male player portrayed her, the ghost vehemently rejects the Tyrant's theatrical representation of her body. Govianus's participation in this representation in order to undo it contributes to a meta-theatrical affirmation of the ability of theatre itself to correct its abusers. On the whole, the Lady's demands on Govianus ultimately link political tyranny to the male usurpation of the female body in a way that pushes him to become a legitimate governor, mainly through recognizing and respecting her authority over herself.

The ghost's silence during her final appearance to accompany her body to its grave, along with Govianus's defensiveness at this last appearance, however, bring back that sense of reserve or dissatisfaction on the Lady's part and guilt on Govianus's. Despite having exhibited the strongest will and discernment, qualities belonging to the soul and making her more effective at governing than Govianus, the Lady ends up as a disembodied soul sombrely following her own corpse offstage like a chief mourner in a funeral procession, while Govianus, who has already failed once to maintain the throne, again enjoys the government of the kingdom. The Lady's ghost's continued attachment to her body challenges the tendency to define the body negatively in opposition to the soul – a tendency that undergirds the cultural commonplace of categorizing women as either carnally or spiritually oriented, whores or saints. The play highlights this commonplace through its structural opposition of the Wife with the Lady, but it also exposes how male attempts to thwart or test the female will, in both plots, ultimately amount to self-destructive tyranny that pushes women to these extremes that have become stereotypes. The final image of the Lady herself literally split into two as she exits the stage literalizes this division of women into oppositional categories in a way that suggests the violence of such dichotomous thinking.

Stone and Spirit in *The Winter's Tale* and *The Duchess of Malfi*

Despite the rarity of female stage ghosts, at least two plays featuring ghostly encounters with female characters, if not actual ghosts, bear striking similarities to *The Lady's Tragedy*. Shakespeare's *The Winter's Tale* (1609–1611) and Webster's *The Duchess of Malfi* (1613–1614), each performed within a few years, at most, of *The Lady's Tragedy*, also portray strong-willed, authoritative, and aristocratic female characters who become disembodied voices. In Shakespeare's play, Antigonus is haunted by a dream vision of Hermione that he suspects was more than a dream. He tells Hermione's infant daughter, before abandoning her in the wilderness on Leontes's orders:

> I have heard, but not believed, the spirits o'th' dead
> May walk again. If such thing be, thy mother
> Appeared to me last night, for ne'er was dream
> So like a waking.[65]

Hermione remains dignified throughout her ordeal of being imprisoned during and after childbirth, separated from her infant, and publicly tried for adultery by her husband, firmly denouncing Leontes's accusations with calm anger and never losing her composure. The ghostly apparition in Antigonus's dreams, however, is a 'vessel' of 'sorrow', hanging her head to the side, 'gasping to begin some speech', weeping so that 'her eyes / Became two spouts', and vanishing with 'shrieks' (3.3.19–36). Like Hermione and the Lady, Webster's Duchess is confident, self-assured, and articulate. When her brother has her murdered, though, she becomes something even less than a ghost. The Duchess's powerful voice, expressing her

---

[65]   William Shakespeare, *The Winter's Tale*, ed. David Bevington, 3.3.15–18. Further references to *The Winter's Tale* cite this edition.

will to 'assay / this dangerous venture' of choosing a second husband despite her brothers' fierce opposition, as well as her strong sense of her own identity and dignity in the face of torture when she asserts 'I am the Duchess of Malfi still', is reduced to a ghostly echo. This echo conveys an unsuccessful warning to her husband – the man she once governed publicly and wooed privately – by repeating the last few words of his sentences.[66] In short, all three assertive, confident female figures end up as disembodied voices in some form or another.

The Duchess's disembodied voice and the fleeting glimpse Antonio catches in 'a clear light' of 'a face folded in sorrow' (5.3.43–4) find a counterpoint in the earlier image the Duchess conjures of a concrete monument, the 'figure cut in alabaster / kneels at my husband's tomb' (1.2.364–5). Similarly, the ghost-vision of Hermione contrasts with the statue of Hermione that Paulina unveils at the end of *The Winter's Tale*, and the Lady's ghost in *The Lady's Tragedy* offsets the marble effigy that forms her tomb, where she first appears to Govianus.

In all three plays that present these oppositional images of the lady as stone and as spirit, the lady is unable to occupy a middle ground between these states of cold, rigid physicality and eerie immateriality. In *The Lady's Tragedy* the Lady's warm physical expression of love for Govianus in the first scene is short-lived – she kills herself with the inflexible view that a forced body will tarnish her spiritual value. For Leontes in *The Winter's Tale*, Hermione simply cannot be a sensual woman, warmly affectionate with her guests, comfortable in her pregnant body, and yet remain chaste. For Ferdinand and the Cardinal in *The Duchess of Malfi*, the Duchess cannot remain virtuous and loyal to them while seeking a second marriage out of personal desire and affection rather than out of duty. Each of these plays shows men obsessively trying to control a woman's body, and a woman attempting to recover the body, at least to some extent, from the damage of this control. Facing murder, the Duchess requests that her body be bestowed upon her women (4.2.220–21). Hermione is concerned with recovering the fruit of her body: when she returns as a statue that comes to life, her first words are not for her repentant husband, but for her daughter, to whom she reveals, 'I, / Knowing by Paulina that the oracle / Gave hope thou wast in being, have preserved / Myself to see the issue' (5.3.126–9). As in *The Lady's Tragedy*, this concern for the body, expressed on the brink of death in one case and seemingly from beyond the grave in another, insists on a more complex understanding of the female self than that imposed by the counter images of stone or spirit.

Is it just a coincidence that these three plays, staged within a few seasons of one another and portraying strong-willed, authoritative women, provide images of those women as both disembodied spirits and stone monuments? The onstage presence of statue figures of the women, or the evocation of such a statue in *The Duchess of Malfi*, perhaps alludes to the story of Pygmalion, who created a stone

---

[66]   John Webster, *The Duchess of Malfi*, ed. Leah S. Marcus, 1.2.262–3, 4.2.137, 5.3.19–44. Subsequent references to *The Duchess of Malfi* cite this edition.

sculpture of his version of the ideal woman – a woman that did not exist in reality.[67] Leontes, Ferdinand, and the Tyrant essentially force their own versions of the ideal woman onto Hermione, the Duchess, and the Lady, and become destructive when the real women before them do not fit into their respective delusions – that a woman cannot be chaste and also friendly to her husband's dearest friend (Leontes), that an honourable woman will have no desire for married love beyond what family duty requires of her (Ferdinand), or that a woman will defer to masculine power defined by conquest (the Tyrant). The men turn the women into stone, literally into the stone of funeral monuments,[68] and figuratively as well in terms of the Lady's stony resolve to kill herself and the stony composure of both Hermione and the Duchess, who, prior to their respective ordeals, were so vibrant and joyfully affectionate. The ghostly visions of the women do offer a thematic contrast with the stone monuments, but these apparently opposite images share a similar function. Both stony and ghostly figures are abstractions of the woman made possible by her violent removal from the sphere of the living, a removal from the possibility of her body and spirit acting together with direct impact on those around her.

Dramatists, of course, draw inspiration from one another's plays, and the similar patterns of stones and spirits, wilful aristocratic women and obsessively controlling men in *The Winter's Tale*, *The Duchess of Malfi*, and *The Lady's Tragedy* might simply reflect this cross-pollination. These plays nonetheless form part of what Hopkins and Liebler have identified as an increased interest in tragic female protagonists, and certainly, while Middleton revisits many of his own thematic concerns from *The Revenger's Tragedy*, among the most significant differences his revisiting offers is that Gloriana now has a voice in her successor, the Lady. The alternate stone and ghost images of captivating female figures destroyed by men who take patriarchal expectations of women to the extreme at the very least encourage a rethinking of those expectations, and in a way that connects ideas about women to understandings of the soul-body, immaterial-material dynamic.

---

[67]   Eaton, 'Seeing the Emblematic Woman', 73, finds that the Tyrant and Govianus of *The Lady's Tragedy* share Pygmalion's perception of women.

[68]   Beyond the Duchess's evocation, early in the play, of the image of a funeral monument in the figure of a kneeling woman, as Leah Marcus (ed.), *The Duchess of Malfi*, 0 sd n., suggests, 'the Duchess's grave may be visible onstage' in 5.3. Marcus also notes that 'the reference to *dead stones* (35) may refer to her grave, as well as to the *ruins* (2), which were probably not represented onstage in early productions'.

Chapter 4
Observer and Spectacle

Ben Jonson refers to the poetry and written record of the masques he produced with Inigo Jones as the 'spirit' that remains long after the masque is over and its courtly participants 'deface' the masque's physical 'carcass' of scenery, costuming, and props.[1] With the dominant presence of Anna of Denmark and her ladies on the masquing stage early in James's English reign,[2] Jonson's repeated comparison of the masque's material and immaterial components to the body-soul dynamic opens another window onto the gendered and political nature of that very dynamic. Anna's performances and the texts surrounding them, I argue, productively unsettle the gender-coded distinctions between body and soul, material and immaterial. This creative revisioning of soul-body ideas makes a claim for women's political relevance, that is, for the importance of women's influence over and contribution to the state and its politics beyond their bodily roles. My first chapter looked at two plays that staged a frustration of the male desire to puppet women, a frustration that resulted from the unmanageable signifying force of feminized onstage material, while my second chapter focused on a play that demonstrated an awareness of the body-soul relationship as a rhetorical construct available for witty manipulation in gender struggles for power. This chapter extends the insights of my first two chapters by interrogating how the silent, performing body of the female masquer itself engages in rhetorical manipulation of the gendered body-soul divide. It also builds on Chapter 3's exploration of female ghostliness as both defusing and symbolizing female authority by analyzing how the masquing female body comes to represent the soul differently – and without the narrative of death and disembodiment.

Current feminist masque criticism moves us away from the view of the court masque as a monolithic expression of the monarch's will, to draw attention to Anna of Denmark's astute political uses of the masque as well as to her influence over its creative development.[3] My chapter adds to the critical work on women's

---

[1]   Ben Jonson, *The Masque of Blackness*, ed. Kristen McDermott, ll. 6–19. All subsequent citations of *Blackness* are to line number in this edition. See also Ben Jonson, *Hymenaei*, ed. Stephen Orgel, ll. 2–9. Subsequent references to *Hymenaei* cite line numbers in this edition.

[2]   Clare McManus, *Women on the Renaissance Stage*, 99.

[3]   See especially Barbara Kiefer Lewalski, *Writing Women*, 15–43, for an exploration of Anna's 'use of the court masque as a vehicle for self-affirmation and for subversive intervention in Jacobean politics'. David Bevington and Peter Holbrook (eds), *Politics of the Stuart Court Masque*, 8–9, write that 'court masque needs to be viewed as a diverse expression of conflicting arenas of interest within court culture, rather than as primarily

contributions to governance and the state through masque performance by combining this area of inquiry with a consideration of masque's thematic and structural engagement with the soul-body dynamic. Masque criticism has not previously joined these two areas of study to the extent that I seek to develop their relationship in this chapter, unless to emphasize a fundamental disconnect between masque's textual definitions of the soul-body divide and the masquers' physical performance. Recent scholarship has indeed helpfully addressed the problematic tendency for critics to privilege the masque writer's published account of the masque despite the fact that these accounts really only represent a fraction of the event, since the bulk of the masque was taken up with various dances for which detailed records and music compositions are not available.[4] Sophie Tomlinson warns, however, that the resulting 'critical focus on the material dimension of the masque has occluded the richness of Jonson's poetic figuring of femininity'.[5] With Tomlinson's point in mind, I posit that Jonson's 'spirit'-'carcass' construction of the masque form is not detached from the reality of performance, where 'the female body' is 'the locus of action and meaning'.[6] Instead, Jonson's text draws attention to the potential for the composite structure of the masque's tangible and intangible elements to engage cultural notions of the body-soul relationship. These notions, as I have been arguing, directly impact representations of and attitudes towards women. Approaching women's political use of the masque and the masque's engagement of body-soul ideas as deeply related offers insight into a form of female transgression other than the threatening display of aggressive sexuality that has, as I discuss further on, attracted critical attention. The transgressiveness I am interested in has to do with women's bodily

---

a symbolic ceremony vital to the reproduction of monarchal power'. They further claim that *The Masque of Blackness* 'shows Jonson and Inigo Jones following the lead of Queen Anne', who used the masque to present herself as 'unmanageable' and to 'establish a new transgressive mode of womanliness, one calculated to arouse masculine anxiety' (11–12). Holbrook, 'Jacobean Masques', 79, discusses *The Masque of Queens* as an expression of Anna's 'views on the worth and dignity of women' and a 'bid for transfer of power from King to Queen'. Leeds Barroll, 'Inventing the Stuart Masque', 121, 132, discusses 'the first Stuart masques as a forwarding of the *Queen's* programmes. As a cultural activity primarily involving noblewomen, these royal spectacles deflected attention from the King and his own circle to focus on the new court of the Queen' and to 'establish a context for the exercise of her own politics'. Other scholars who attend to Anna's political uses of masque and her influence on its creative development include Clare McManus, Stephanie Hodgson-Wright, and Sophie Tomlinson.

 [4]   Leeds Barroll, *Anna of Denmark*, 84, for instance, finds it needful to 'correct the imbalance resulting from critical emphasis on the *word* by shifting the analytical focus to the masque's five distinct stages of organization', four of which 'comprised activity not expressed or expressible in words alone'. See also McManus, *Women on the Renaissance Stage*, 18.

 [5]   Sophie Tomlinson, *Women on Stage*, 25.

 [6]   Lewalski, *Writing Women*, 30.

representation of the soul – an entity that was most often masculinized through its contradistinction from a feminized body. Combining these two areas of inquiry also leads me to think of dance in a new way. Building on critical discussion of early modern dance as a physical mode of communication, I consider dance as an activity that bridges corporeal movement and abstract thought, body and soul. Dance is not only central to masque, but central to masque's engagement with the gendered soul-body divide.

The Soul of the State

As courtly art form and entertainment, the masque itself functioned more broadly as a representation of the 'soul' of the state, or of the moral condition of the state's governing power, its monarchy. The scriptural injunction that a wife submit to her husband just as the body submits to the head and the church submits to Christ, which I discuss in Chapter 2, mapped easily onto the model of a king's position in relation to his subjects.[7] The subjects form the body politic that the king governs as its head, which is synonymous, of course, with the intellect, chief faculty of the soul. In fact, insofar as Christ rules the 'kingdom' of heaven, and the divinely appointed king claims his authority to rule from Christ, the parallel relationships between Christ and church, and king and subjects, merge. To give only one example of the pervasive mental associations between these overlapping hierarchies, Thomas Adams describes how 'in man there is a kingdome … The mind hath sovereignty over the body', and he locates this kingdom 'within' as the first in an echoing series of kingdoms that progresses from man over beast to husband over household, magistrate over community, king over realm, and, finally, God over everything.[8] By analogy, then, the state's governing power equates with its 'soul'. Indeed, Jonathan Goldberg claims that James 'was the soul of the masque' along with Jonson's poetic invention.[9] And yet the masque, as courtly entertainment designed to celebrate and affirm the monarch's 'natural' and benevolent ruling power at the pinnacle of a divinely ordained hierarchy, could also reflect the health of the 'soul' and moral guide of the state in critically suggestive ways. Stephen Orgel asserts that although as a genre masque 'is the opposite of satire', with its harshly corrective aims, it still holds the capacity to educate and persuade through a strategic use of praise.[10]

---

[7] Ephesians 5:23: 'For the husband is the head of the wife, even as Christ is the head of the church: and he is the saviour of the body'.

[8] Thomas Adams, *The Workes of Tho: Adams*, 431.

[9] Jonathan Goldberg, *James I*, 58.

[10] Stephen Orgel, *Illusion of Power*, 40.

Masque Structure and the Soul-Body Analogy

Masque as a genre foregrounds the physical and the dancing body through elaborate and extravagant scenery and costume, and yet relies on poetry to convey and preserve the eternal virtues and ideals that the spectacle represents. In this way, the genre engages a conceptual physical-spiritual divide on the level of structure. Jonson, the most prominent masque writer at the onset of James's reign, draws attention to this divide. In its capacity to advise on and reflect the moral condition of the body and soul of the state, masque extends this structural and thematic concern outward. While as performers and collaborators[11] women formed a part of the masque's structural and thematic engagement with the body-soul dynamic, then, their masque participation also held potential to critically reflect on the state.

How might the dance performance of female masquers comment on the governance or 'soul' of the state, however, when pervasive cultural stereotypes, supported by contemporary religious and medical ideas, associated women with the body and therefore prescribed and justified their subjection to men, contrastingly associated with reason? Jonson's masques frequently stage the decisive triumph of perfect virtue, reason, order, and aristocratic decorum over vice, unruly passion, chaos, and bodily impropriety, making it clear that King James, the privileged spectator to whose gaze the entire masque is subject, is the ultimate source of the triumphant forces.[12] Can the silent, aristocratic female masquers move beyond a puppet-like signifying of the monarch's benevolent power when the 'female body' itself was 'subjugated to the monarch's will within the discourse of courtly

---

[11]   The queen and her ladies became involved in a masque's development long before final rehearsals. Jonson himself acknowledges Anna as the source of important artistic decisions (such as, for instance, the ladies' appearance in blackface in *Blackness* and the inclusion of an anti-masque in *Queens*); Jones presented preliminary costume sketches to Anna for her approval and adjustments; ladies had a say in their own costumes and appearance, and as Lewalski, *Writing Women*, 28, notes, may even 'have offered other suggestions as the masques took shape'. Stephen Orgel, 'Marginal Jonson', 151–2, offers evidence of women's involvement in their costume decisions. At first 'puzzled by the fact that Jones regularly did his costume designs in monochrome ... and indicated the colours with annotations', Orgel discovered that 'Jones would do his designs, and submit them, with his suggestions, to the Queen. She then chose the colours, and made whatever changes in the design that she wished'. Orgel, 153, also describes an illustrative instance of Lucy Harrington, countess of Bedford, depicted wearing a single skirt for *Hymenaei* (1606), when Jones's original design called for a double skirt. 'That is the way this aristocratic dancer preferred to appear', Orgel explains; 'she paid for the costume, and her own dressmaker made it. The other dancers would have felt entitled to make their own alterations in their costumes as well'.

[12]   On this pattern, see Stephen Orgel, *Illusion of Power*, 40; Holbrook, 'Jacobean Masques', 71; and McManus, *Women on the Renaissance Stage*, 120. According to Goldberg, *James I*, 59, the king 'sits observing and yet informing the masque', and is 'the moving power of its invention'. For more on James as the ultimate source and enabler of the masques, see Goldberg, *James I*, 62–5.

magnificence'?[13] As I discuss in previous chapters, early modern humoural theory held that women were more vulnerable than men to the type of unruly passions and irrationality that Jonson's masques stage James's kingly power as conquering. With reference to *Titus Andronicus*, *Hamlet*, and *Cymbeline*, moreover, Susan Dunn-Hensley discusses how Shakespeare frequently 'links the rampant, uncontrollable sexuality of the queen with the world of nature, and ... the chaotic world of nature and sexuality threatens to disrupt the ordered world of politics'.[14] Katherine Eggert also discusses anxiety over female rule, noting that 'Renaissance culture viewed women, usually with great suspicion, as inherently changeable and hence unreliable'.[15] How might female masquers' bodies resist their connection to political disruption and instability while challenging James's authority as 'soul' of the state in order to make a claim for women's relevance to state politics?

James himself is clear on his view that women have no place in politics. In his advice on kingship addressed to his son, for instance, James gives counsel on how Prince Henry should treat his future wife:

> And for your behaviour to your Wife, the Scripture can best give you counsel therein. Treat her as your owne flesh, command her as her Lord, cherish her as your helper, rule her as your pupil, and teach her in all things; but teach her not to be curious in things that belong her not: Ye are the head, shee is your body; it is your office to command, and hers to obey ... [S]uffer her never to meddle with the Politicke government of the Common-weale, but hold her at the Oeconomicke rule of the house; and yet all to be subject to your direction.[16]

For James, the conventional appeal to the hierarchy of head over body serves not only to legitimize a husband's pre-ordained authority over his wife, but also to bar women from participation in the politics of government.[17] Just prior to this passage, James emphasizes how a future king's marriage to an infertile woman would constitute a disaster to the commonwealth, effectively underscoring that the most important political contribution the queen can ever make is a bodily one – the production of heirs.

---

[13] McManus, *Women on the Renaissance Stage*, 120.

[14] Susan Dunn-Hensley, 'Whore Queens', 102.

[15] Katherine Eggert, *Showing Like a Queen*, 4–6, 21.

[16] James I, *Basilikon Doron*, 173. See Ch. 1 of Lewalski's *Writing Women* for a discussion of James's lack of success in imposing these particular views on Anna, and on the Protestant clergy's attempts to frame her role in a similar way.

[17] Eve is another biblical source for women's subjection to their husbands and concomitant exclusion from political affairs. While 'the most burdensome and wide-ranging effect of the malediction of Eve is the subjection of women to their husbands', Ian Maclean, *Renaissance Notion of Woman*, 2.9.1, observes that 'it is also inferred from the subordination of Eve that woman should not play any part in the running of the state or in public affairs, but should occupy herself with 'woman's work'.

Jonson's division of the masque into 'spirit' and 'carcass', as Clare McManus interprets this division with its attendant 'value-judgement', seems to agree with James's relegation of women to their bodily roles in that, according to the logic of Jonson's analogy, the female masquers, who were 'denied access to spoken text', belong firmly to the 'carcass' of the masque production.[18] Like the 'music for which no text survives', or the 'scenery and costume' whose designs Jonson did not include in his publications, the 'movement of the body, both danced and unchoreographed', had 'no textual representation' and so was destined to fade away with the rest of the ephemeral (and by implication inferior) physical elements of the performance.[19] McManus asserts, however, that 'Jonson's framing statement offers a theorisation of the masque' that is simply 'not available in performance', where the silent but expressive female body, and not the poetry of the masque, commanded the audience's attention.[20] Samuel Daniel attests to this reality in the preface to *The Vision of the Twelve Goddesses* (1604), the first masque Anna performed in, when he comments on the practicality of poetically describing the goddesses (Anna and her ladies) *before* their entrance onstage, because otherwise 'the eyes of the Spectators' might 'beguile their eares, as in such cases it ever happens, whiles pomp and splendour of the sight takes up all the intention without regard what is spoken'.[21] The centrality and signifying power of the performing female body in Anna's masques might overshadow the written and spoken text, and yet this prominence of the body does not leave the 'spirit' half of the familiar divide behind so as to make Jonson's spirit-carcass theorization of the masque on paper 'unavailable' in performance, as McManus would argue. I suggest, by contrast, that masque performance evokes ideas of the soul-body dynamic as they intersect with representations of women, and it does so in a way that pushes against the conventional hierarchy of soul over body that is readily available to Jonson as a means of privileging the component of the masque for which he was responsible – its poetry.

Even Jonson's equation of the masque's poetry with its 'spirit' and its physical apparatus with its 'carcass', however, is not a straightforwardly hierarchical division. Certainly a sense of the superiority Jonson attributes to the immaterial and enduring written word over the masque's short-lived material beauty comes through in the assertion that 'little had been done to the study of magnificence in these [masques]' – that is, no one would be interested in these events – if their 'spirits' had 'perished' with the dismantling of the masque's physical trappings

---

[18]   McManus, *Women on the Renaissance Stage*, 10.

[19]   Ibid.

[20]   Ibid. Indeed, McManus, 99, reminds us that inevitably, 'in a culture accustomed to transvestite male performance, and within which the staging of the female body was a rarity not legitimately witnessed beyond the confines of the court community, tensions surrounded the performance of the aristocratic female body'.

[21]   410. All citations of *Twelve Goddesses* refer to page numbers of the 1623 edition in *The Whole Workes of Samuel Daniel*.

(*Blackness*, 10–14). Jonson later emphasizes what he calls the 'noble and just advantage' of 'things subjected to understanding' over things 'objected to sense' in the wedding masque *Hymenaie* (1606):

> the one sort [things objected to sense] are but momentary and merely taking, the other impressing and lasting. Else the glory of all these solemnities had perished like a blaze and gone out in the beholders' eyes. So short lived are the bodies of all things in comparison of their souls. And, though bodies ofttimes have the ill luck to be sensually preferred, they find afterwards the good fortune, when souls live, to be utterly forgotten. (2–9)

Again, Jonson makes clear the superiority of the 'spirit': anything perceived through the senses is 'but' momentary and 'merely' taking. That bodies have the 'ill' luck to be sensually preferred implies a value judgement that they should not be preferred, and their 'good' fortune in finally being forgotten while souls live on likewise conveys the sentiment that bodies should be forgotten. An underlying note of sarcasm might also be present in these lines, expressive of derision for the body and its fate. And yet, in spite of this devaluing of and even contempt for the (masque) body, Jonson frames the 'spirit', his writing, as existing for and because of the body: he writes, here, precisely so that the 'glories' of the masque 'solemnities' will not perish 'like a blaze' and go out 'in the beholders' eyes'. The body of the masque, to put it differently, is the predicate of this writing. Similarly, in *The Masque of Blackness* (1605), Jonson presents his writing as performing a 'duty' to 'that majesty that gave [the masques] their authority and grace', and as aiming to 'redeem' the 'solemnities' from 'ignorance' and 'envy' (14–19). His description, moreover, of the courtly audience tearing down the masque's scenery after the performance as a 'defacing' allowed by their 'privilege' presents the destruction of the scenery as a wasteful and almost violent act that his writing attempts to mitigate, and not as the deserved fate of an inferior portion of the production (*Blackness*, 12–13). While Jonson's language undeniably elevates 'writing' and 'spirit' over the masque's 'carcass', then, his invocation of the soul-body dynamic as a means of understanding masque structure also permits ambiguity, leaving open the possibility for conflicting interpretations.[22]

---

[22]   Thomas M. Greene, 'Ben Jonson and the Centered Self', 326, observes an ambiguity in Jonson very similar to the ambiguity I am identifying here. He discusses Jonson's characteristic emphasis on the symbols of the circle and its centre, representing 'harmony and completeness ... stability, repose, fixation, duration'. 'The associations of the circle – as metaphysical, political, and moral ideal, as proportion and equilibrium, as cosmos, realm, society, estate, marriage, [and] harmonious soul', Greene explains, 'are doubled by the associations of a center – governor, participant, house, inner self, [and] identity' (326). Jonson usually privileges the ideal of the complete circle and what Greene calls the 'centered' or 'gathered' self, a self defined by inner stability, self-reliance, and stillness. And yet at times Jonson indulges in a 'kind of witty complicity' with 'his disguisers' 'in spite of himself' (336). His 'disguisers' represent a more 'protean' or 'chameleon' self that succeeds better than a fixed self 'in the disoriented world of Jonson's comedies', a world where 'the

In his preface to *Tethys Festival* (1610), Samuel Daniel inverts the value that Jonson attaches to the writing of masques in comparison to their physical performance. Daniel ends his preface with the assertion that:

> in these things [masques] wherein the only life consists in shew: the arte and invention of the Architect gives the greatest grace, and is of most importance: ours, the least part and of least note in the time of the performance thereof.[23]

Not only does Daniel hold his written 'part' to be barely noticeable during performance, but as a writer he counts himself among 'the poore Inginers for shadowes' who 'frame onely images of no result', adding that 'our greatest knowledges' are not 'fixt' but 'rowle according to the uncertaine motion of opinion, and controwleable by any surly shew of reason' (E1v). In Daniel's juxtaposition of his writing with the architectural masque art of Jones, writing is the insubstantial and secondary element attempting to 'shadow' with images 'of no result' the primary, concrete images that by implication are 'of result' or have a greater initial impact on their audience. Writing is not spirit-like here in terms of its enduring quality; rather, its immateriality translates into a lack of consequence. Daniel's very different construction of writing connects with an unusual disparagement of 'reason' as 'double edged': it 'strikes every way alike', and 'when al is done', 'understanding' remains 'subject to al passio[n]s & imperfections' (E1v–E2r). Daniel presents reason as fallible in this way in order to insist, as part of his pre-emptive address to future critics of his publication, that no one is entitled to pass judgement as if his[24] reasoning ability were better than anyone else's, or as if it were exempt from the influence of the passions. Daniel's strategy to avoid censure groups 'reason' (chief faculty of the soul) with writing, and downplays these while acknowledging the greater impact of the 'passions' (usually associated with the body) and the physical architecture of the masque. This strategy underscores the relevance of the body-soul dynamic as a means of understanding masque structure. Both Jonson and Daniel conceptualize their masques in terms of this dynamic, even while taking up clashing critical positions on the role of each element.

---

outer circle is broken' (336–7, 326). The world of the 'uncentred and misshapen' circle is a world of 'flux or … mobility, grotesquely or dazzlingly fluid' (326). In this world, a self that is too rigidly isolated fails, as *Epicoene*'s Morose exemplifies (335). Greene notes that 'to sketch these categories [i.e., circle and incomplete, off-centre circle] is to seem to suggest absolute poles, ethically positive and negative. But although much of Jonson's writing encourages that suggestion, it does not lack its tensions, its ambivalences, its subtle shifts of emphasis' (326). The tension that Greene perceives between 'centripetal' and 'centrifugal' images, that is, between durability and changeability, corresponds, I think, to the ambiguity inherent in Jonson's seeming privileging of the permanent 'soul' of masque over its more ephemeral body.

[23]   Samuel Daniel, *Tethys Festivall*, in *The Order and Solemnitie of the Creation of … Prince Henrie*, E2r. Subsequent citations of *Tethys Festival* refer to this edition.

[24]   Daniel is explicitly addressing male readers in this passage.

Embodying Wit in Queen Anna's Masques

In female performance the location of the female body within masque structure can suggest an alternative to the dismissive and delimiting cultural association of women with the body, an association that excluded women from official involvement in politics. Even though McManus is correct in pointing out that, according to the logic of Jonson's spirit-carcass theorization of masque form, female masquers belong to the 'carcass' part of the event,[25] Jonson himself seems to locate performers outside of this analogy. In *Hymenaei* he follows his comments on the difference between soul and body (analogous with 'things subjected to understanding' and 'those ... objected to the sense') with the claim that:

> This it is hath made the most royal princes and greatest persons, who are commonly the personators of these actions, not only studious of riches and magnificence in the outward celebration or show, which rightly becomes them, but curious after the most high and hearty inventions to furnish the inward parts. (9–14)

Here, Jonson credits those who participate in and commission the masque with recognizing the importance of the 'inward parts' in relation to the 'outward celebration', and with a resulting desire for both components to achieve 'magnificence'; he does not present the participants as themselves constituting the outward parts.[26] Likewise, Daniel's division of the written from the physical masque, 'images of no result' from images of result, is clearly a division between two art forms – his own and that of 'the Architect', Inigo Jones; bodies are not an explicit part of the equation (E2r). Instead, masquers' dancing bodies disrupt the equation. They bridge the categories of the masque's 'carcass' and 'spirit'. The dancing bodies are silent and physical along with the masque's set, but self-moving as opposed to mechanical, and as persuasive and communicative in their movements as the masque's words (if not more so, according to Daniel's avoidance of setting his text in competition with the entrance of the queen and her ladies). By placing the body in a liminal position between the masque's structural 'carcass' and 'spirit', masque permits the body itself to escape its own physicality and the values attached to the physical in contrast to the spiritual.

In support of the body's liminal position within masque structure, I turn to the early modern association between dance and speech. If dance functions as a recognizable language for the body, then the body is not a mere material instrument to convey the meaning in the poetry of the masque's narration, but a producer of its own text. Even Jonson, who takes the position that the dancing bodies carry

---

[25] McManus, *Women on the Renaissance Stage*, 10, 37.

[26] Similarly, in *Blackness*, when Jonson describes the masque participants as exercising their privilege 'to deface their carcasses', he is speaking of their practice of dismantling the masque's scenery; they do not, of course, deface themselves. Again, Jonson does not group the masquers' bodies with the masque body.

out 'the author's' 'invention', admits that dance can cause confusion about the real source of meaning. He recalls a segment in *Hymenaei* in which the masquers

> danced forth a most neat and curious measure, full of subtlety and device, which was so excellently performed as it seemed to take away that spirit from the invention which the invention gave to it, and left it doubtful whether the forms flowed more perfectly from the author's brain or their feet. (279–83)

Adding to this doubt is the construction of dance as a form of rhetoric in early modern dance treatises. In *Orchesography* (1588), Thoinot Arbeau calls dance a 'dumb rhetoric by which the orator, without speaking a single word, can, by virtue of his movements, make the spectators understand that he is gay, worthy to be praised, loved and adored'.[27] To uphold his claim that 'dancing is a manner of speech',[28] Arbeau provides the examples of 'the daughter of Herodias who obtained what she demanded of King Herod Antipas after she had danced', and of 'Roscius', who 'moved the spectators' through 'gestures and mime' 'as much as Cicero had been able to do by eloquence of his orations, or even more'.[29] Here, dance is more powerful than speech as a form of persuasion – a radical possibility for women masquers when decorum prohibited their verbal performance on stage. Thomas Elyot's *The Boke Named the Governour* furnishes another example of dance as speech that is explicit about dance's subversive potential. When the 'cruel tirant' 'Niero' perceived his people's 'hatered' towards him and feared 'lest by mutuall com[m]unication they shulde conspire agayne him', he prohibited words, dictating that gestures replace speech. When these gestures eventually 'grewe to a perfecte and delectable dauncinge', Niero 'at the laste was slayne of his people moste miserably'.[30] Again, the understanding of dance as a communicative tool, in this case to resist political oppression that centred on the restriction of speech, could lend radical implications to the dance of female masquers led by a queen whose views frequently opposed the king's.

Though less concerned with political implications, John Davies's treatment of the connection between dance and speech exemplifies how this connection problematizes any definition of dance as strictly physical. In Davies's poetic celebration of dance, 'Orchestra' (1596), Antinous presents speech itself as a dance of the air:

---

[27]   Thoinot Arbeau, *Orchesography*, 23. In John Davies's 'Orchestra', 93, Antinous inverts Arbeau's claim that dance is a form of rhetoric by instead claiming that the art of rhetoric is itself a form of dance, or rather, adds complexity to the dance that speech itself constitutes.

[28]   McManus, *Women on the Renaissance Stage*, 38, finds that Arbeau's 'comparison of the dance's steps to a linguistic grammar … makes the systemic nature of this communicative code and its independent generation of meaning explicit'.

[29]   Arbeau, *Orchesography*, 23.

[30]   Thomas Elyot, *Boke Named the Governour*, fols 77–8.

For when you breath, the ayre in order moves,
Now in, now out, in time and measure trew;
And when you speake, so well she [the air] dauncing loves,
That doubling oft, and oft redoubling new,
With thousand formes she doth her selfe endew:
    For all the words that from your lips repaire,
    Are nought but tricks and turnings of the aire.[31]

While we might read the swirling dance of air as presenting speech in physical terms,[32] reading these lines as extending the act of dance beyond the visibly material to the immaterial is equally plausible. This plausibility finds support in Antinous's assertion – immediately following his claim that 'beauty' and 'love' dance in all Penelope's body parts, her 'pulses' and 'vaines' – that 'all the vertues' that 'flow' from Penelope's 'soule' also form a 'measure', a 'Daunce' which Antinous cannot 'conceive' with his eyes.[33] Just as speech itself amounts to a dance, 'Logick leadeth Reason in a dance', according to Antinous, in that 'with close following and continuance / One reason doth another so ensue' in a dance-like formation conforming to logic's guidance.[34] 'Orchestra' presents dance, then, as an activity that does not belong strictly to the body, but involves the unseen – speech, breath, the soul, reason – as much as the physical.

While scholars agree on the connections between speech and dance[35] in early modern thought, they diverge in their interpretations of the significance of this connection. Skiles Howard argues that 'courtly dancing was not only an aspect of elite culture related to linguistic forms, it was a discursive practice in its own

---

[31]   Davies, 'Orchestra', 44. The notion of speech as itself a dance also appears earlier, in stanza 25:

the Queene with her sweet lips divine
Gently began to move the subtile ayre,
Which gladly yielding, did it selfe incline
To take a shape betweene those rubies fayre
And being formed, softly did repayre
With twenty doublings in the emptie way,
Unto *Antinous* eares, and thus did say.

[32]   McManus, *Women on the Renaissance Stage*, 38, adopts this reading. With reference to the stanza I quote in the note above, she comments: 'In asserting speech's physicality, this passage also reinforces the contemporary association between feminine speech and sexuality'.

[33]   Davies, 'Orchestra', 105–8.

[34]   Ibid., 94.

[35]   Besides its connection to oratory, the 'connection of dancing with writing', and with poetry in particular, 'was a Renaissance commonplace', and Skiles Howard, *Politics of Courtly Dancing*, 22, reviews various examples, such as Thomas Morley's explanation of the galliard through reference to the trochaic foot in verse. Davies, 'Orchestra', 65–70, also likens dance steps to poetic feet when he compares dance 'measures' to 'Spondeis', galliards to pentameter, corantos to dactyls, and lavoltas to anapests.

right', and as such had 'power both to circulate social norms and to negotiate new formations'.[36] With particular attention to the female masquing practice of tracing letters or forming symbols through dance patterns, a practice which 'intensified the interaction of dance and language', McManus draws attention to the 'legibility of the body, and of the female body in particular' in masque, exploring the tensions between the dancing body as a passive, 'legible' object of interpretation and an active agent of expression.[37] Whereas McManus focuses on how the 'text' of the female masquers' performance often opposes or complicates the meaning that the published text imposes on the dancing body, Sophie Tomlinson points out instances where the particular expressiveness of the female dancing body and particular lines in the written masque text could perfectly complement each other.[38] I want to add to these rich interpretations of early modern dance's connection to speech a reading that takes into account the significance of dance not only as a physicalized form of speech[39] but as an activity that, as Davies shows, was thought to bridge physical movement and non-physical thought, body and soul. In this capacity, dance, the central component of masque entertainment, is also central to my consideration of the intersection between representations of women in masque and early modern ideas of the soul-body dynamic.

Bodily 'speech' in masque performance, of course, comes in different forms. Critics have pointed out how female masquers' overtly sexualized appearance threatened to subvert conventional gender hierarchy. Orgel notes that the revealing costuming of Anna and her ladies in *Blackness* that Dudley Carleton famously criticized as 'too light and courtesan-like' was objectionable because it was 'too blatantly feminine, but also, in its aggressive display of sexuality – Queen Anne was visibly pregnant – paradoxically masculine as well'.[40] McManus underlines the connection between 'public female speech and a dangerously liberated

---

[36]   Howard, *Politics of Courtly Dancing*, 22–3.

[37]   McManus, *Women on the Renaissance Stage*, 36–43.

[38]   Tomlinson, *Women on Stage*, 22–3.

[39]   McManus, *Women on the Renaissance Stage*, 15–17, emphasizes dance's significance as a physicalized form of speech.

[40]   Orgel, 'Marginal Jonson', 149–50. Orgel, *Impersonations*, 110, also notes that in *Queens*, 'the fearsome and the admirable share the same attributes of masculine vigor, strength and independence – the witches are the queens in reverse, literally, etymologically "preposterous" ... [T]he witches, defining themselves as "faithful opposites / To fame and glory", *produce* their heroic antitheses ... And ... it is precisely the masculinity of the queens that constitutes their virtue: they are not Elyot's "mild, timorous, tractable" creatures, but armed and aggressive'. Even though 'man-like and unseemly clothes', such as those Anna wears in Paul van Somer's 1617 portrait of her, could 'be an index to a much more dangerous kind of independence', Orgel also attends to the similarities between fashions worn by men and women (84–100). He stresses, more generally, the need to rethink 'the gender assumptions of English theatre history on the basis of ... evidence' that women were not categorically excluded from early modern English stages, as critics tend to assume (1–9).

female sexuality in the open display of the gendered body' by citing Francesco Barbaro's claim in *On Wifely Duties* that 'the speech of a noble woman can be no less dangerous than the nakedness of her limbs'.[41] In contrast to this transgressive potential of the body's 'speech', McManus also emphasizes, along with Bella Mirabella, that courtly dance inscribes restrictive social codes onto the body and that participation in public dance amounts to an enactment and affirmation of those codes.[42] While I agree with these readings, I posit that the masquing female body could also 'speak' transgression beyond appearing aggressively sexual and could, even while acquiescing to codes of gender and social hierarchy as these codes were built into the formalities of courtly dance, undermine a fundamental conceptual support for those hierarchies – the gendered concept of the soul-body divide. In several masque performances, the female body, far from serving as the usual counterpoint to 'masculine' reason, visually and thematically comes to signify the soul, with subversive implications for traditional gender relationships, implications that align with the political statements Anna communicated through her masque involvement.

Masques, as Daniel, Jonson, and Jones developed the form under Anna's patronage,[43] visually juxtaposed bodies with scenery. Even though Jones mechanized the elaborate sets so that the scenery itself was impressively mobile, both moving and stationary parts of the set provided a structured framework that would offer contrast to the fluidity of the masquers' bodies, a fluidity that both dance

---

[41]   McManus, *Women on the Renaissance Stage*, 6. Barbaro's claim predates *Blackness* by almost 200 years but, as McManus asserts, it 'remained representative of prevalent attitudes which governed opportunities for women's performance in the early seventeenth century; the danger of the female voice and body is powerfully constant'.

[42]   McManus, *Women on the Renaissance Stage*, 8, discusses how 'dance's social nature opened it to the female performer and sought to mark her as an acquiescent member of courtly society; dance training formed part of the literal incorporation into the individual of the controls exerted upon the noble body. The noblewoman's danced participation was intrinsic to the masque genre ... for it to offer the social affirmation necessary to its existence as state ritual'. McManus, 25–6, also describes 'the reverence, or bow' at the beginning of each dance as 'a gesture of respect to the dance partner, which, when performed to the monarch, was also an expression of the sovereign's elevated status' and so 'a bodily affirmation of the social order'. 'When men and women of the Renaissance danced', Mirabella, 'Mute Rhetorics', 413, notes, 'they played out their assigned social and psychological roles in their dance steps'.

[43]   'When Jonson says that he "apted" his invention to the commands of Queen Anne in writing *The Masque of Blackness*', Orgel, 'Marginal Jonson', 153, observes, 'he is acknowledging that his poetic invention follows, depends upon, and is subject to the authority of the Queen; the conceit of blackness is the Queen's. If we took the patronage system seriously, the Queen's invention would be as interesting to us as Jonson's'. McManus, *Women on the Renaissance Stage*, 98–9, notes that 'the fluidity of the staging of the female body found in the distinct approaches of [Daniel's *Twelve Goddesses* and Jonson's *Masque of Queens*] ... ties them to the masque career of Anna of Denmark'. On Anna's creative influence, see also Lewalski, *Writing Women*, 28.

and costume emphasized. This contrast visually invokes the body-soul dynamic in a way that aligns the female body with the soul. Explicit verbal references to the body-soul dynamic in masques, such as the River Niger's comparison of the 'mixture' of bodies and souls to the mixture of fresh water and brine in *Blackness* (115–20) or Iris's description of the queen's and her ladies' bodies as 'Temples' that receive the spirits of goddesses in *Tethys Festival* (420), invite the audience to perceive this further, visual invocation of the body-soul relationship. A song in Daniel's *Tethys Festival* even expresses confusion as to whether the 'figures' we see are 'shadowes' or 'bodies', and advises the audience to 'Take' the 'Glory' of the sight 'sodaine as it flies / Though you take it not to hold' (F3v). The intangible, evanescent 'wonder' of the dancing bodies here evokes the soul, which, though eternal according to Christian belief, was also characterized as the body's temporary guest, and often pictured in its fleeting moment of departure.[44]

Tethys Festival, a masque in which Anna performed at the celebrations for Henry's creation as Prince of Wales, strikingly exemplifies the juxtaposition of fluid bodies with more rigid, stationary scenery. Two 'great' statues 'of twelve foot high', representing Neptune and Nereus, receive first mention in Daniel's description of the masque's opening scene (E2v–E3r). 'These Sea-gods', Daniel relates, 'stood on pedestals and were al of gold', with 'pilasters' behind them, which 'bore up a rich Freeze' to form a frame for the initial 'harbour' scene. Against the framework of this imposing statuary, 'Eight little Ladies' perform their dance around the young prince Charles (impersonating Zephyrus) (E3v, F1r). Their 'light robes adorned with flowers, their haire hanging downe, and waving with Garlands of water ornaments on their heads' convey their fluidity as 'Nymphs of fountaines' (E3r–E3v). The subsequent scene, featuring the grand revelation of Anna and her ladies, amplifies this initial juxtaposition of feminine fluidity with decidedly masculine statuary. Queen Anna and her ladies, as Tethys and her nymphs of English rivers, appear enthroned in five 'Cavernes'. Concave shapes feature prominently in this second set, including not only the separate caverns and the shape of the set as a whole (it 'came into the forme of a halfe round') but also the bowls of several fountains, 'out of which issued aboundance of water' (F1v–F2v).[45]

Combined with the notion that Tethys and her river nymphs 'invest[ed]' the bodies of Anna and her ladies (F4v), the scenic emphasis on concave, water-bearing shapes would seem to foreground the notion of woman as vessel, as 'bearer of significance' rather than producer of significance.[46] But if the masque invokes this association, it more persuasively disrupts it. As river nymphs, the women

---

[44]   Rosalie Osmond, *Imagining the Soul*, gathers several illustrations of the soul. For medieval and early modern examples of the soul depicted in its moment of departing flight, see illustrations VIII, 7, 27, and 31.

[45]   When describing the first fountain, Daniel notes that it used 'artificiall water' (F1v).

[46]   McManus, *Women on the Renaissance Stage*, 10, 16, also discusses the female masquers' challenge to this stereotype.

descend from their structured caverns 'with winding meanders like a River' to present their offerings at the 'Tree of victory' (F2v). Their attire complements this fluid mobility: it includes a 'waving' veil, 'upper garments' of 'sky-coloured taffetas for lightnes', 'halfe skirts' with 'the grou[n]d work cut out for lightnes', and a 'long skirt ... wrought with lace, waved round about like a River' (F2v). The alignment of women not with the scene's prominent vessels, but with their contents, the flowing water, associates them with active significance and mobility. For Stephanie Hodgson-Wright, the women's representation of rivers and the sea, the 'most valuable geographical features of a pre-industrial country', is a means of claiming 'socio-economic importance'.[47] Lewalski finds that in representing Tethys and the ocean, Anna 'claims as her own' an 'alternative sphere of power and worth' to that of James, and 'embodies the quintessentially female waters of the oceans and rivers, with all their wealth and peaceful industry'.[48] Both these readings point out that the masque's presentation of women as watery nyads connotes female self-assertion and agency. These empowering connotations, I posit, are very much connected to an alternative view of the gendered soul-body dynamic, in that the alignment of women with water here links to an alignment of women with the soul, both constrained by and yet resisting the constraint of the enclosing 'body' of the set.

The gendering of that constraining 'body' as masculine completes the reversal of the usual gendering of the body as feminine and the soul or reason as masculine. Neptune and Nereus, figures of male kingship and industry, are immobile statues, aligned with the passive stone of the great fountains in contrast to the dancing women aligned with the 'spouting water' (F2v). Neptune's trident carries over to the two great tridents framing Tethys's throne, whose symmetry further echoes Neptune's and Nereus's positioning at either side of the first scene. While these symbols of masculine authority frame Tethys and define her own position of authority, she and her ladies descend freely from the set's framing structure to present their offerings at the tree of victory. Before her appearance, Tethys/Anna also makes gifts, through her messenger, of a trident to James and a sword and sash to Henry. As a gift, the trident is as much an 'ensigne' of Tethys's 'love' as of James's 'right' to rule, while the sword, derived from a female authority, 'Astraea', comes with instructions: it must not be 'unsheath'd but on just ground', and must be kept with the scarf of 'love and Amitie', a scarf that figures forth the extent of the empire Henry will inherit, the limits of which he is forbidden to 'passe' (E4v–F1r). Rather than constituting a willing affirmation of male authority to govern, then, these gifts present women as both enabling and circumscribing that power. Visually, this female self-assertion under the guise of accepting the monarch's

---

[47] Stephanie Hodgson-Wright, 'Beauty, Chastity and Wit', 44.

[48] Lewalski, *Writing Women*, 40. The 'quintessentially female' quality of the waters that Lewalski perceives is something positive here, opposing the tendency to pathologize and disparage women's bodies and tongues as overly 'leaky', which Gail Kern Paster has investigated.

'right' to rule corresponds to the women's 'winding' movement within, and yet in stark contrast to, the framing and masculinized set of tridents, pillars, and statues.

The Masque of Queens (1609) features a similar pattern – evocative of the body-soul divide – of fluid female movement out of a more rigid structure associated with masculine authority. In this masque, Queen Anna and her ladies portray famous warrior queens whose stories appear in established literary and historical canons, as Jonson's extensive marginal notes attest. They first appear enthroned in the House of Fame, a 'glorious and magnificent building' with 'Men-making poets' for 'columns', as well as columns made of the men those poets wrote about.[49] This striking image of women framed within male literary tradition (the House of Fame itself comes from Chaucer [494]) figures forth how, in McManus's words, the masque limited women to 'their representation' in 'male-authored texts', showing them as 'written about rather than writing' and 'subject to the authority of the male canon'.[50] The masquers' departure from this structure, then, becomes loaded with meaning. McManus's insight into the masque's variation of 'the gendered premises of Renaissance architecture' points to an inversion like that in *Tethys Festival*. *Queens* turns the 'female caryatid', which normally 'bore the building's physical weight', into 'an embellishing female statue, free to descend from Jones's elaborate pedestal'. Conversely, the 'male body', which usually bore the 'conceptual weight' of the 'architecture's aesthetic and ideological standard', in *Queens* becomes the 'passive' bearer of physical weight.[51] As in *Tethys Festival*, the framing structure of the set, with its clearly defined shape, is masculinized and contrasts with the fluid dance movements of the female masquers' bodies. The masquers might start out as embellishing statues, but, excepting Anna, they all represent dead historical figures who live 'eternised' in the House of Fame, and are 'visible' for just this night (403, 419). They represent spirits, in other words, which adds to the masquers' fluid, ethereal quality. The use of male professionals to portray the 'hags' in their excessive carnality sets off the 'real' female bodies of the queens as comparably less carnal and further underlines the masque's association between physicality and masculinity. McManus describes the House of Fame in terms of 'containment' and 'restrictive boundaries' that the masquers negotiated and 'finally abandoned' to 'generate significance through movement in the masquing dance (social and performative) on the floor of the Banqueting House'.[52] All these elements – the positioning of women's dancing bodies as a vibrant, moving, 'signifying force'[53] in contrast to the comparably passive, less mobile scenery, the characterization of the women as spirits only

---

[49]   Jonson, *The Masque of Queens*, ed. Kristen McDermott, ll. 375–8. Further references to *Queens* are to line number of this edition. Homer, Virgil, and Lucan formed some of the House's columns, for instance, as did Achilles, Aeneas, and Caesar (487–92).

[50]   McManus, *Women on the Renaissance Stage*, 112.

[51]   Ibid., 117.

[52]   Ibid., 117–19.

[53]   Ibid., 117.

briefly perceptible, and even the dancers' expansive emergence out onto the dance floor from within the bones or pillars of the House – visually evoke the soul-body dynamic.

In these evocations, women align with the soul insofar as early modern thinkers often conceptualize the soul as the active principle, responsible for thought (signification) and movement, and see the earthly body as the bearer, the frame, and often the limiting cage for the soul (though it is a cage the soul will eventually escape). Francis Quarles's eighth emblem in book 5 of his 1635 *Emblemes* exemplifies the continuing currency of the notion that the body encages the soul.[54] This emblem (see the cover illustration of this book) shows a fully fleshed human figure praying behind bars – that is, inside the ribcage of an oversized skeleton. Besides the concept of body-as-cage, the illustration also exhibits the tendency to visually depict the soul as a body. If a cultural alignment of women with the body and of men with reason could be so disadvantageous to women, justifying and naturalizing male authority to govern them, what might these masques say about that male authority in visually reversing the usual alignment to present masculine restraint over women as similar to the body's restraint over the soul? Through their evocation of the soul with fluid dance mobility alongside masculinized framing structures, do female masquing bodies engage in a visual rhetoric questioning the authority for that restraint? The body might confine the soul, for instance, but not because of an inherent authority within the body itself or out of a need to keep the soul in check. Instead, a failure of body and soul to cooperate and balance each other leads to an unproductive impasse, as seventeenth-century body-soul dialogues make clear.[55]

Such a critique of the restrictions men imposed on women would likely be welcome to Anna, whose own views about her self-worth apart from her connection to James,[56] and about her role as queen, frequently clashed with James's position that women had no place in the affairs of government and naturally owed obedience to their husbands. Scholars including Barbara K. Lewalski, Leeds Barroll, Clare McManus, and Sophie Tomlinson have documented specific instances of Anna's use of the masque, and other means available to her, to make political statements that often opposed James's absolute authority as husband and monarch. Anna selected her ladies-in-waiting and principal co-performers, for instance, not according to the political prowess of their male relations, but according to her own esteem for the individual women.[57] She used the 'taking-out' moment in masque (when the dancers select partners from the courtly audience) to honour

---

[54] Francis Quarles, *Emblemes*, 272.

[55] On the unresolved incompatibility between body and soul in seventeenth-century body-soul dialogues, see Osmond, *Mutual Accusation*, 97–101.

[56] Anna insisted on her royal identity as independent from her marriage to James, emphasizing her own family's lineage and her position in the Danish royalty. See Lewalski, *Writing Women*, 16–19.

[57] Barroll, 'Inventing the Stuart Masque', 124–5.

male individuals of her choosing, without constraining herself or her ladies to James's personal favourites.[58] Anna's invitations to the masque sometimes caused problems for James with an offended French ambassador when she favoured the Spanish ambassador as an indication of her own 'support for Spanish Catholic interests'.[59] Anna patronized the Children of the Queen's Revels, an acting company frequently reprimanded for satire against James, which may indicate her own enjoyment of such satire.[60] Leveraging a political situation to her advantage in her vehement opposition to James on a family matter – his decision to remove Henry to the guardianship of the earl of Mar – Anna refused to accompany James to England for his succession to Elizabeth until Henry was returned to her.[61] While her earlier military attempt to retrieve Henry was unsuccessful, this time James succumbed to her demands in order to avoid the political embarrassment of entering England with his consort noticeably absent.[62] One of the most explicit instances of Anna's interest in politics and her confidence in her own governing capabilities is her earnest – but ultimately ignored – desire to reign as regent in London during James's 1617 progress to Scotland.[63] This brief review of some of Anna's politically charged actions demonstrates that within the masques she played a key role in developing, a visual rhetoric of the body which subverts the usual gendering of body and soul in order to represent women more advantageously

---

[58]   Ibid., 129–31.

[59]   Lewalski, *Writing Women*, 29. Another possibility is that having Anna carry the blame for the Spanish ambassador's invitation to, for instance, *The Masque of Beauty* was useful for James. Appearing towards the French ambassador 'extremely sorry for the inconsiderateness of the Queen' may have been part of James's strategy to honor the Spanish ambassador at the masque while avoiding or lessening, as much as possible, offense to the rival French ambassador, as Mary Sullivan explains in *Court Masques of James I*, 37–43. If this was James's strategy, however, it involved acknowledging Anna's power of political interference (the king had to admit that he could not override the queen and uninvite the Spanish ambassador to please the French), and it left James open to the French ambassador's observation that he was not 'master in his own house' (Sullivan, 37). For more on the political significance of masques and the vying between the French and Spanish ambassadors for invitations, see Sullivan, 1–82.

[60]   Lewalski, *Writing Women*, 24.

[61]   Ibid., 20.

[62]   Ibid.

[63]   Clare McManus, 'Memorialising Anna of Denmark's Court', 84. McManus, 84–9, describes how, when James bypassed Anna to appoint Francis Bacon as 'nominal head of state' along with the Archbishop of Canterbury, Anna retaliated, in a sense, by giving audience, in her own court, to a ladies' masque that her favourite, Lady Bedford, commissioned for her. We can read Anna's occupation of the privileged position of chief observer, reserved in every other Jacobean masque for James, as a means of symbolically and publicly reaffirming her own authority and capability of governing in the position that James denied her, as McManus has convincingly argued.

would accord well with Anna's self-promotion and with her valuing of women independently from their connections to men.

Nonetheless, as Lewalski remarks, 'we need not suppose contestation and subversion to be fully conscious on the Queen's or the authors' parts' for the subversion to be present.[64] So far I have focused on *Tethys Festival* and *The Masque of Queens* to develop my point about the visual alignment of women with the soul through the juxtaposition of bodies with scenery, but women consistently represent immaterial figures in Anna's masques. Before *Tethys Festival*, in *The Masque of Blackness*, the ladies' apparel as water nymphs, with its layered, flowing, and transparent materials, also emphasized the fluidity of the nymphs and their movements. *The Vision of the Twelve Goddesses* asks us to see the bodies of Anna and her ladies as making visible the spirits of goddesses (414). Night and Slomber insist on the immateriality of these 'Figures of the light' by making it clear from the outset that they will appear to the courtly audience in a dream that Slomber will induce (413–14). When female performance onstage was a novelty not yet possible on the commercial stage,[65] then, the courtly women who could be physically present on a formal stage through masque redefined their physicality, using it to stand in for the spiritual and immaterial. In part, the personification of abstract ideals and virtues, often in the form of divine figures from classical myth, is simply a characteristic of the masque genre, which aimed to glorify the monarch as the source and perfect embodiment of such virtues.[66] Nonetheless, we should not neglect the creative influence Anna had on the development of the genre, including her idea to have the anti-masque in *Queens*, which had the effect of offsetting the ethereal physicality of the female masquers with the excessive corporeality of the hags that professional male actors represented.[67] And again, regardless of intention or female direction in this case, masque's immaterial figures

---

[64] Lewalski, *Writing Women*, 29.

[65] In *Women on Stage*, Ch. 1, Tomlinson discusses female masque performance as an important precedent that connects to and influences eventual female performance on the commercial stage.

[66] See for instance, *Queens*, 415–22:

> She [Anna] this [honour conferred by the 11 dead queens] embracing with a virtuous joy,
> Far from self-love, as humbling all her worth
> To him that gave it, hath again brought forth
> Their [the queens'] names to memory; and means this night
> To make them once more visible to light,
> And to that light from whence her truth of spirit
> Confesseth all the lustre of her merit:
> To you [James], most royal and most happy king.

[67] The juxtaposition of bodily vice in the anti-masque with ideal virtue in the masque recurs in later masques, perhaps most explicitly in *Pleasure Reconciled to Virtue*, and continues as a theme much later, in Townshend's *Tempe Restored*, for instance, and Milton's *Comus*.

carried special significance for female performance because of the usual gendering of material and immaterial.

Whether or not it was deliberate, the masque's overturning of the common gendering of the soul-body divide underlies and supports what Lewalski identifies as the masque's subversion of 'the representation of James as exclusive locus of power and virtue by means of texts and symbolic actions which exalt the power and virtue of the Queen and her ladies – and, by extension, of women generally'.[68] Above, I cite the masquers' activity and movement (in contrast with the less mobile scenery that both frames and bears the weight of the masquers) as qualities aligning them with the soul. Helkiah Crooke describes the soul as 'incorporeal and diffusive, quickening, sustaining, governing, and moving the whole body'.[69] The explicit connection Crooke sees between 'moving' and 'governing', here, is part of what makes the representation of women as aligned with the soul an empowering one. Because of the soul's conventional role as governor of the body, in visually associating women with the active soul, these masques decentre James as having the sole prerogative to rule, and challenge the notion that men are the only ones capable of contributing, intellectually, to affairs of government, while women are relegated to bodily roles of child-bearing and -rearing. In *Tethys Festival*, Triton even calls 'mightie Tethys' the 'intelligence' that governs the ocean (or 'moves the Sphere / Of circling waves') (E4r). If, moreover, masque is a reflection of the soul or moral health of a state, the very representation of women as the active, moving 'soul' or centre of Anna's masques implies that women are likewise central – and not just in a bodily way – to the state's well-being.[70]

---

[68]   Lewalski, *Writing Women*, 29. Lewalski suggests that this subversion results from 'the need to please multiple audiences – King, Queen, male courtiers, court ladies – and from the complexities of shared authorial responsibility with the Queen-patron'.

[69]   Helkiah Crooke, *Mikrokosmographia*, Bk. 1, p. 2. More examples of the view that movement signals the soul's presence appear in Simon Harward, *Discourse Concerning the Soule*, fol. 7, 9, which cites Aristotle's definition of the soul as the 'continued motion' of the 'organicall body' and lists 'voluntary motions' as part of the rational faculty of the soul according to Plato's division of the soul's three faculties. John Woolton, *Immortalitie of the Soule*, fol. 5, also cites Aristotle as the source for the notion of the soul as '*the first Action or the continuall motion of a body organicall*' and categorizes 'movement' as a property of the rational soul according to Plato's theory. William Hill, *Infancie of the Soule*, C1r, D2r, E2r, repeats the reference to Plato and Aristotle as authorities for the position that the soul is the body's 'first moover', and refers to a pregnant woman's experience of an unborn child moving within her womb as support for his claim that infants in the womb possess a soul.

[70]   Greene, 'Ben Jonson and the Centered Self', 326–7, finds that 'the great storehouse of Jonson's centripetal images is the series of masques which assert, almost by definition, the existence of an order'. With specific reference to *The Masque of Beauty*, Greene claims that the 'choreographed' and 'poetic' 'circles of the masques have reference first of all to the central figure of the king, literally seated in the center of the hall and directly facing the stage area. The king, associated repeatedly with the sun, is himself a symbolic orb – fixed, life-giving, dependable'. For Greene, 'the king's presence opposite the masquing stage … represents a kind of metaphysical principle which the dancers attempt to embody'.

Even while dance is communicative and active, it also poses a potential problem for the visual reading of the female masquers as aligned with the soul, in that conventionally, women's dance parts were passive and served to set off their male partners' more complex and showy dance steps. A woman's 'dance steps were smaller, lower to the ground, delicate and not rambunctious or too energetic', signalling that she 'deferred to [her partner's] assumed greater talent and presence'.[71] Pointing out that men were the dance masters, choreographers, and writers of dance music and dance manuals, Mirabella argues that 'dance was constructed to put women on display for those in power, for the male patriarchy', and that 'dancing women, their movements under constant surveillance, were controlled and restrained'.[72] Mirabella focuses on how dance 'support[s] male power' through the dynamics of the gaze, noting that women were not supposed to 'return the man's gaze': 'downcast eyes is the recommended behaviour for women in the Renaissance, and the dance masters are very clear on this point'.[73] This dynamic between gazer and object of the gaze (the active gaze implying dominance and control, and the passive reception of the gaze implying submission) is especially relevant to a masque setting in which the king enjoyed a prominent seat of honour in the audience and, supposedly, the best sightlines.[74] We might identify the moment in which female masquers entered the audience to choose dance partners as an instance of female agency that breaks the power dynamic

---

I am suggesting a different possibility here, namely, that the female dancers themselves represent 'a kind of metaphysical principle'. Visually, they also form the dynamic centre of the masque structure as viewed from the audience – an alternate centre that stands in competition to James as centre of the hall. (The notion that the masque functions as mirror to the audience further supports the idea of twin, competing centres, as I discuss further on in this chapter). Greene, 330–33, argues that Jonson's ideal of being centred does not necessitate physical rootedness, but rather involves moving and acting always according to one's moral anchor. Thus, as much as James is a moral centre that the masquers reflect, the masquers themselves signify a moral centre for James and the state to reflect. In light of Greene's insights, the women's appearance as a moral centre need have nothing to do with physical confinement within the domestic sphere.

[71] Mirabella, 'Mute Rhetorics', 425.

[72] Ibid., 415. See also McManus, *Women on the Renaissance Stage*, 55: 'The representation of dance in contemporary literature robbed the eroticised female dancer of agency, fetishising her and privileging the male author and dancer. ... Despite the necessity of women to the dance, theirs was a marginal and physical presence. Eloquently expressing her distance from representation, the female dancer was reduced to a bodiless hand at the edge of an illustration [in Arbeau]. Such strategies of exclusion were embodied in other dance manuals in rather more subtle ways than in Arbeau's, concentrating instead on the management of the female body'.

[73] Mirabella, 'Mute Rhetorics', 424–5.

[74] McManus, *Women on the Renaissance Stage*, 42–3, points out that in some instances the spectators in the less privileged seats in the galleries enjoyed the better perspective – as when the figures or patterns formed by dancers were likely easier to discern from above.

of the gaze, but Davies seems to explain away this possibility in stanza 112 of 'Orchestra':

> What if by often enterchange of place
> sometime the woman get the upper hand?
> That is but done for more delightfull grace,
> For on that part shee doth not ever stand:
> But, as the Measures law doth her commaund,
>> Shee wheeles about, and ere the daunce doth end,
>> Into her former place shee doth transcend.

For Mirabella, Davies here shows 'how successfully dance functioned to maintain and enforce femininity' when he 'reassures himself' that even if dancing 'might allow women some freedom and the chance to get the "upper hand"', it will soon 'right the situation and put the woman back in her place'.[75] The reassurance that Mirabella perceives in Davies's passage, however, also marks, without entirely dissolving, an underlying anxiety about the possibility of a woman's brief dominance within dance.

The unease evident in Davies's need to emphasize the temporariness of women's potential dominance in dance also surfaces in treatises like Elyot's, which took pains to define the proper demeanour for a female dancer. With tactics like 'lasse advauncing of the body', she must balance her male partner's 'naturall' 'fiercenesse' with 'mildenesse', his 'Audacitie' with 'timerositie', his 'wilfull opinion' with 'Tractabilitie', etc.[76] The very effort to provide guidelines suggests that courtiers did not necessarily take these dance attitudes for granted or fall into such attitudes naturally through their supposed knowledge of 'all qualities incide[n]t to a man and also ... to a woman'.[77] Without dismissing the real obstacles that dance decorum based on conventional gender ideology posed to female masquers' expressions of assertiveness, we can read this concern to control or limit forms of dance expressiveness as indicative of the real possibilities dance opened up for challenging gender codes. Barbara Ravelhofer objects to applying concepts of 'the "active male gaze" and its "passive" female counterpart on the complex interaction of dancing', on the grounds that 'certainties gained from the safe distance of a text or image appear less evident once the practical implications of actual movement come into play'.[78] The passive demeanour that writing on dance recommended for female dancers, then, did not necessarily diminish an emphatic liveliness and energy on the part of Anna and her ladies, framed within the confines of the masculinized scenery.

The female masquers' alignment with the soul through active movement corresponds with female agency in the masque's narratives and helps to reconfigure

---

[75]   Mirabella, 'Mute Rhetorics', 424.

[76]   Elyot, *Boke Named the Governour*, fol. 83.

[77]   Ibid.

[78]   Barbara Ravelhofer, *Early Stuart Masque*, 118.

the motif of possession or puppetry. Puppetry, as I discuss in Chapter 1, often gendered the passive material vessel or puppet as feminine, and the possessor or puppeteer as masculine.[79] Daniel makes divine possession an explicit part of the narrative in both *The Vision of the Twelve Goddesses* and *Tethys Festival*. In *Tethys Festival*, Triton informs the audience that in returning to her 'watery mansion' after several dances, Tethys and her company (played, of course, by Anna and her ladies) will 'shift those formes, wherein her power did daigne / T'invest her selfe and hers, and ... restore / Them to themselves whose beauteous shapes they wore' (F4r). Anna and her ladies are not merely 'shapes' that Tethys and her nymphs 'wore', according to this account. Instead, their 'shapes' are distinguished from 'themselves', in that Tethys's departure restores the ladies' 'shapes' (the referent of 'them') to their 'selves'. More important, the departure of goddess and nymphs does not leave behind diminished shells or rob Anna and her ladies of any splendour: with the reappearance of the queen and her train 'in figures of their owne', the audience is treated to a 'transformation of farre more delight / ... then can be / Discrib'd in an imaginary sight' (F4r). Daniel's choice of the word 'invest' to articulate the deities' presence in the masquers' bodies is also significant. Insofar as 'invest' meant 'to put on as clothes or ornaments', it coordinates with the notion of goddess and nymphs 'wearing' the shapes of courtly ladies, but 'invest' also carried a figurative sense: 'to clothe or endue with attributes, qualities, or a character'.[80] This sense that the goddesses impart their divine qualities to the women, rather than controlling them, comes through in the masque. The first action of Anna and her ladies upon their reappearance is to 'march up to the King ... in a very stately manner' (F4v). This direct advancement to the throne recalls the earlier progression of Tethys and her nymphs when they 'march up' to present floral offerings at the 'Tree of victory' beside the throne (F2v), and the text emphatically presents this earlier progress as expressive of female will. Tethys 'daignes' to appear 'in glory' at Prince Henry's investiture (F3r); she 'resolves t'adorne the day / With her al-gracing presence'; and she comes with a train of nymphs 'she pleas'd to call away' (E4r–E4v). The song lyrics foreground Tethys's gracious choice to honour James, Henry, and the day's event; she is not motivated by obligation, but by her own desire to express 'The vowes [of] her heart' (E3v). The repeated stately advance of Anna and her ladies confirms that the active will of Tethys and her nymphs carries over to the ladies as 'themselves'. The motif of divine animation here, instead of constructing the feminine as passive vessel, empowers the female masquers by highlighting their similarity to the divine force that inhabits them in the masque's narrative – a divine force that in this case is also feminine.

---

[79] For more on the connection between dance movement and female agency in the masques, apart from my focus on puppetry, see Sophie Tomlinson, *Women on Stage*, 19–21, 30–31, 33, 36–7.

[80] *OED*, 'invest', I.1.a. *trans.*, 3. *fig.* a.

The Vision of the Twelve Goddesses similarly presents Anna and her ladies as temporarily possessed by the spirits of female deities and paradoxically stages this possession as empowering for the 'possessed'. At the masque's end Iris describes how 'these divine powers ... cloathed themselves' in the 'appearances' or 'coverings' of Anna and her ladies. But in the dedication to the countess of Bedford preceding the masque text, Daniel makes it clear that 'her Maiestie chose to represent' Pallas, signalling that Anna is really the one who leads her ladies in appropriating the figures of the goddesses in order to present themselves in a particular way before the court (419–20, 407). The masque identifies Anna's chosen goddess as 'the glorious Patronesse of this mighty Monarchy' – that is, as a powerful help and support to the monarchy if respectfully appealed to (420). Again, the masquers' descent from a scenic structure (the mountain) corresponds with active feminine will. After expressing surprise that the goddesses would 'visit this poore Temple', for instance, the prophetess Sybilla remarks that such 'Powers ... shine where they will' (415). If the goddesses' visit to the 'Temple' of the masque hall is somewhat surprising (414), however, their choice to visit the bodies of Anna and her ladies, that is, the 'best-built-Temples of Beauty and Honour', comes across as only natural – a choice undertaken for the goddesses' own 'delight' (420). And while Iris prepares Sybilla and the audience to be overcome by the sight, 'bereave[d] ... of all, save admiration and amazement', the female prophet figure (though a speaking part here performed by a male actor) is not entirely powerless; rather, she prepares the 'Rites' necessary to properly honour the approaching deities and occupies the privileged position of seeing and describing the goddesses through a magic 'Prospective' before anyone else can see them (414–15). As for Anna and her ladies, they do not appear as overcome by the goddess figures but as sharing a lasting affinity with them; their own physical appearance, which the goddesses borrow, is what Iris expects to strike wonder in beholders. At the close of the masque Iris explains that:

> in respect of the persons under whose beautifull coverings they have thus presented themselves, these Deities will be pleased the rather at their invocation (knowing all their desires to be such) as evermore to grace this glorious Monarchy with the Reall effects of these blessings represented. (420)

The goddesses will lend their virtues to England 'in respect of' or for the sake of Anna and her train, or perhaps even through Anna and her ladies, as the referent of 'at their invocation' is ambiguous – 'their' could refer to the goddesses or to the ladies as themselves. Together, the goddesses encompass the power to govern (Juno); wisdom and martial strength (Pallas); diplomacy and peace (Venus and Concordia); virtue (Vesta and Diana); wealth (Proserpina); good judgement (Astraea); and so on (415–17). This statement makes a claim, then, for Anna and her ladies as essential to the monarchy's well-being, not peripheral to its power.[81]

---

[81]   In part, Flora and Ceres, also portrayed in the masque, represent contributions of childbearing and -rearing, though they also stand for a non-physical fertility of 'virtue' and 'beauty' (417).

The idea that the masque serves as a mirror in which the king and audience might see themselves extends the female masquers' active role beyond the fiction of the masque narrative. Where critics have observed 'legible' female bodies to be interpreted by the dominant gaze of the monarch,[82] for instance, we might also observe a performance that aimed to turn that gaze back upon itself – an active reflection of the gaze, instead of a passive subjection to it. In a later masque, *Love's Triumph through Callipolis* (1631), Jonson asserts that 'all representations, especially those of this nature in court, public spectacles, either have been or ought to be the mirrors of man's life, whose ends … ought always to carry a mixture of profit with them no less than delight'.[83] Goldberg takes the position that the spectacle of the masque and the spectacle of the observing king are mirror images that 'bear a single meaning'.[84] Another possibility is that as a mirror, the masque is not simply one with the king's mind, but reflects the monarch with a difference, whether it be a subtle suggestion or even a hint at a flaw. This possibility is more in keeping with early modern uses of the looking-glass metaphor in literary and theatrical contexts beyond the masque. Constructions of theatre and literature as a looking glass for the soul, exposing imperfections with the aim of correcting them, for instance, appear in early modern satire, comedy, devotional poetry, and moral treatises.[85] And even though masque does not operate in the mode of satire

---

[82]   McManus, *Women on the Renaissance Stage*, 39.

[83]   Ben Jonson, *Love's Triumph through Callipolis*, ed. Stephen Orgel, 1–7.

[84]   Goldberg, *James I*, 57. Orgel, *Illusion of Power*, 43, claims that masque form 'was an extension of the royal mind', as does Goldberg, who writes that masque 'represents the king' and 'mirrors the royal mind' (55–7). See also Jerzy Limon, *Masque of Stuart Culture*, 74, on the masque as mirror: 'Jonson considered these highly illusionistic and certainly nonmimetic spectacles "mirrors of man's life". What he actually means is that the laws that govern this artistic reality are by analogy the same as those governing the microcosm of man (who governs his body in the same way as the king his nation), the geocosm of earth, and the macrocosm of the universe'.

[85]   Jonson's *Every Man Out of His Humour*, ed. Helen Ostovich, Induction 20, 116–19, provides an obvious example through the playwright and actor figure, Asper, who announces his intention 't'unmask' 'public vice' by 'oppos[ing] a mirror' to the audience, 'As large as is the stage whereon we act, / Where they shall see the time's deformity / Anatomized in every nerve and sinew'. I. Lada-Richards, '"In the Mirror of the Dance"', 346–7, draws attention to another excellent example in Thomas Randolph's *The Muses Looking-Glasse*, 'a theatrically argued seventeenth-century defence of plays and players in which Roscius, chief actor and master of ceremonies, proclaims the comic stage a mirror for the audience's soul'. Roscius calls 'comedy' the only 'glasse' in which 'the soul sees her face'. Non-dramatic literary works also frequently employ the trope of literature as a mirror for the reader's soul. See, for instance, *The Poems of Aemilia Lanyer*, ed. Susanne Woods: 'To the Queenes Most Excellent Majestie', 37–44; 'The Authors Dreame', 210–12; 'To the Ladie *Margaret*', 27–34; and George Gascoigne, 'The Steele Glas', which sets up his writing as offering an honest reflection of inner truths (within society and within people's characters) in contradistinction to the crystal mirror which flatters with pleasing superficial reflections.

or comedy to correct vice and folly by exposing it to ridicule and scorn, Orgel points out (as I cite earlier in this chapter) that through the very different mode of praise, masque could aim to promote desired behaviour. The masque dancers, furthermore, could perhaps lay special claim to the masque's mirroring function. I. Lada-Richards identifies the 'dancer as mirror' metaphor in Lucian's *De Saltatione* as 'the most important Graeco-Roman pedigree of the "mirror of drama" analogy that dominates the complex theatrical optics of the Medieval and Renaissance European stages'.[86] In theory, then, masque's representation of women as central to the state's political and moral health could prompt in the audience members – through turning their gaze back upon them – a revaluing of their own views on women's roles in state affairs. *Tethys Festival* reflects the gaze quite literally in images that mirror James sitting in state. 'The main visual feature of the masque', Hodgson-Wright asserts, 'is Anna enthroned with her daughter Elizabeth at her feet, a mirror image of the prime spectators, James and the heir apparent'.[87] For Hodgson-Wright, Anna's counter-image foregrounds 'the separateness and femaleness of Anna's court',[88] but it also provocatively opposes the image of James and Henry with a competing female image of monarchy. Tethys might be wife to the 'Oceans King', Oceanus (the name by which her messenger addresses James), but here she appears enthroned alone, facing 'Oceanus' with an image of female majesty that rivals his own (F3r, E4v).[89]

   This mirroring of the king's gaze finds complement in a repeated emphasis on reciprocity in *Tethys Festival*. Tethys's symbolic gift of the trident to Oceanus/ James, as noted above, connects Oceanus's 'right' to rule with Tethys's 'love' – an indication that her acceptance and approval are necessary to validate that right. Tethys's/Anna's gift to Henry, symbolizing his future entitlement to a kingdom, stakes a claim that that 'gift' comes from his mother as well as from his father, and then (as noted earlier) makes clear her expectations that in receiving such a gift, Henry will honour her political advice. The masque introduces this theme of reciprocity earlier on, when Triton fulfills a 'charge' from Tethys 'to say, that even as Seas / And lands, are grac'd by men of worth and might, / So they returne their favours' (E4r). Reciprocity receives similar emphasis in *Twelve Goddesses*. When Anna and her ladies descend from the mountain to deliver 'their presents', actors representing the three graces sing lyrics focusing on the back-and-forth pattern of 'Desert, Reward, and Gratitude' (418). In this masque, the goddesses are the ones who decide on and reward merit, and Sybilla's role, on behalf of 'the Soveraigne

---

   [86]   Lada-Richards, 'In the Mirror of the Dance', 335.

   [87]   Hodgson-Wright, 'Beauty, Chastity and Wit', 44.

   [88]   Ibid., 45.

   [89]   Goldberg, *James I*, 57, describes the masque as a 'mirror' that 'elucidates the spectacle that the king presents sitting in state. The mysteries of the masque reflect the monarch's silent state: the masque represents the king'. The mirroring in *Tethys Festival* elucidates the spectacle of the king in state as a spectacle that need not be masculine by definition, but is equally effective and plausible in feminine form.

and his State', is to properly honour the goddesses with gratitude for their gifts (419). Critics have pointed out that the goddesses' gifts – representing 'armed policie', 'felicitie', 'Justice', and 'power by Sea', among other ideals – imply that these benefits did not exist previously in James's reign.[90] Instead, they arrive from divine (female) sources, and they arrive through women. Ultimately, the masque's mirroring action makes a similar point in that the idealistic reflection of James's rule as blessed with 'true zeale', 'concord', 'plenty' (419), and so on is also a reflection that transposes women onto the centre of the picture.

Although the masquing, dancing female body mirrors the gaze of the monarch and courtly audience, this mirroring does not involve any erasure or concealment of the performers' gender. Instead, a sense of privileged access to the divine through the feminine pervades *Twelve Goddesses* and *Tethys Festival*. These and other masques insist on the role of female physicality as a means to the spiritual.[91] Jonson's decision to have the masquers in *Blackness* approach the audience holding fans marked with 'hieroglyphics' illustrates this insistence (254). Early modern thinkers saw the hieroglyph, McManus explains, as 'eras[ing] the gap between sign and signifier and ... offer[ing] what Bath terms a "natural, Adamic language"'.[92] The masque's hieroglyphs, for McManus, 'attempt to constrain the female to a single, predetermined and readily available authorial meaning, and to limit further the generation of significance through an apparently clear and

---

[90] Lewalski, *Writing Women*, 30; Hodgson-Wright, 'Beauty, Chastity and Wit', 43.

[91] Mary Floyd-Wilson, *English Ethnicity and Race in Early Modern Drama*, 125–7, asserts that the female masquers' physical appearance signifies *internal* virtue in her compelling argument about *The Masque of Blackness*'s complex engagement with the pressing political and cultural anxieties over James's desired union between Scotland and England. 'Jonson portrays the Ethiopians' complexion not only in terms of the western aesthetics of "great beauty's war"', she explains, 'but also as a temperament associated with the inner qualities of wisdom, civility, piety, constancy, and a contemplative nature'. Floyd-Wilson suggests that 'the deferred transformation of the Ethiopians' skin – from black to white – is only one half of the masque's imagined exchange: Britannia promises external whiteness, but gains the internal qualities of a black complexion ... Britain not only receives the Ethiopians' hieroglyphs, it absorbs their humoral qualities into its land and water – the very humoral qualities that should remedy the northerner's spongy nature and dull wits'. (The essay explores the masque's fascinating 'geohumoralism' that sees the Ethiopians' environmentally influenced humours as balancing the humours of the 'barbaric' Northerners – the Scots and Picts – and so enhancing the union of England and Scotland.) Floyd-Wilson further demonstrates a link between the physical mark of unchanging blackness and the spiritual purity to which Niger lays claim when he speaks of his fresh stream as able to mingle uncontaminated with the ocean's salt water, just as the soul mingles with, but is uncontaminated by, the body. 'The nature of that uncorrupted substance is alluded to', Floyd-Wilson claims, 'when Jonson calls the Ethiopian nymphs "Daughters of the subtle flood" ... "Subtle" humors are those which have achieved a thin, rarefied state, and the subtle qualities of Ficinian/Aristotelian ... black bile are what produce genius in a person's body'.

[92] McManus, *Women on the Renaissance Stage*, 14.

available representation of what was defined as the feminine essence'.[93] While McManus acknowledges that the actual female performance thwarts this authorial 'attempt' at exact definition, that the masque indeed presented 'qualities of grace and fertility and spiritual beauty' through 'female corporeality', she perceives a fundamental conflict between the ideals signalled by the hieroglyphs (as dominant ideology defined those ideals) and the 'open display of the gendered body' (again, as dominant ideology would define it – sexual and threatening).[94] But evoking, through the hieroglyph, the idea of a perfect, direct language with the elimination of any gap between sign and signifier, or between physical form and abstract ideal, also makes a point about the female body as simultaneously the physical form and abstract ideal. This implication demands that we look beyond the initial tension between physical and ideal to see how their union, in the hieroglyph of the female body, necessitates a redefinition of both the ideal term and its physical representation. For instance, in *Blackness*, the hieroglyphs Anna bears on her fan indicate the name 'Euphoris' (meaning 'abundance'[95]) and the symbol of a 'golden tree laden with fruit' (261–2). Where McManus conceives a 'destabilising' incompatibility between the women's bodies as 'markers of a dangerous and open sexuality'[96] and the connotations of spiritual fertility, generosity, and purity in this and other masquers' symbols, we might also perceive an assertive reclamation and redefinition of the exposed female body as something beyond the purely sexual – as something, in other words, deeply connected to spiritual abundance and generosity as signalled by the hieroglyph and its function.

The notion that the physically present female masquers are themselves realizations of the ideal, that rather than illustrating or bearing meaning they constitute the meaning, also comes into play in *Twelve Goddesses*. Preparing the audience for the ladies' entrance, Iris describes how the goddesses choose to 'appeare' just as 'antiquity hath formerly cloathed them', explaining that 'the imagination of piety' has cast 'the gifts and effects of an eternall power' in 'mortal shapes' to render them comprehensible. She adds that 'mortall men' have also given 'that shape wherein themselves are much delighted' – the shape of a woman – to 'all the Graces', 'Blessings', and 'Vertues' (414). This passage betrays how the conventional feminizing of abstract virtues is caught up with a sense of male control: 'men' have actively 'apparelled' blessings, virtues, and the graces with the shapes of women in order to procure their own visual delight and to render such 'mystical Ideas' more available, manageable, 'easier to be read' (414). This dynamic closely relates to the widespread tradition of envisioning the soul as a beautiful woman.[97] In her extensive study of historical imaginings of the soul,

---

[93]   Ibid.

[94]   Ibid., 6, 15.

[95]   McDermott, *The Masque of Blackness*, 205.

[96]   McManus, *Women on the Renaissance Stage*, 15.

[97]   Osmond, *Imagining the Soul*, 47, reminds us that 'the word "soul" itself is feminine in Greek, Latin and all romance languages, German, and even Arabic'.

Osmond concludes that mainly male artists are behind the construction of the soul as a woman.[98] As with depicting abstract ideals and virtues as female figures, envisioning the soul as a woman provides a measure of control over – a means of grasping, of containing – the concept of the soul. The image of the soul as a woman rarely appears in pointed opposition to a masculinized body and carries little mitigating force for the cultural assumption that real women were in general more bodily creatures compared to men, who were supposedly more rational. That men could express admiration for a woman's strong intellect by claiming she had a 'manly soul'[99] speaks to the detachment of the image of the soul-as-woman from attitudes towards real women, or in other words, to its status as little more than a dead metaphor, a convention worn out to the point of meaninglessness.

Female masquing performance, however, could reinvigorate the image of the soul as a woman. In *Twelve Goddesses*, male control over what can 'best represent the beautie of heavenly Powers' ends abruptly with the appearance of Anna and her ladies, as Daniel signals with his explanation that Iris must describe the goddesses before they enter because their 'presence' takes away speech (414–15). In impersonating goddesses who epitomize specific ideals and virtues, such as Pallas ('Wit and Courage') or Vesta ('Zeale' and 'Purity'), Anna and her ladies reclaim these virtues and powers from feminized abstractions to qualities that real women – and especially women – possess. As Hodgson-Wright observes, 'although Anna and her ladies are playing parts, it is their very likeness to those parts which makes their representation successful',[100] and indeed, Iris relates how the goddesses have chosen to manifest themselves through the queen and her ladies because, as the 'best-built-Temples of Beauty and Honour' (420), they provide the best fit. In *Tethys Festival*, the reappearance of the ladies as 'themselves' immediately following their dance as Tethys and her nymphs underscores the sameness between the real women and the goddesses known for their individual virtues. The link Iris makes between 'beauty' and 'honour' here fits into a consistent thematic connection

---

[98]   Ibid., 47. Osmond explores some of the historical and cultural roots of this tradition throughout Ch. 2.

[99]   Ben Jonson, 'Epigram LXXVI: On Lucy, Countess of Bedford', p. 128, l. 13. Jonson's compliment to Bedford, Anna's favorite, contrasts her 'softest virtue … / Fit in that softer bosom to reside', with her 'many soul' that should 'control' 'with even powers, / The rock, the spindle, and the shears' – objects that represent both the fates and female domestic authority (11–15). For another example, see Davies's 'Orchestra', stanza 68, which describes the galliard as:

A gallant daunce, that lively doth bewray
A spirit and a virtue Masculine,
Impatient that her house on earth should stay
(Since she her selfe is fierie and divine)
Oft doth she make her body upward flyne.

Here, though Davies assigns feminine pronouns to the soul, he characterizes the attributes and expressions of the soul as 'masculine'.

[100]   Hodgson-Wright, 'Beauty, Chastity and Wit', 44.

in Anna's masques between beauty and virtue more generally. Hodgson-Wright suggests that 'Anna and her ladies ... create a female presence upon the stage by claiming beauty as innately feminine, a quintessential quality not easily imitated by male actors'.[101] She cites as one example the triumph of the queens over the hags in *Queens*: instead of reading the hags' defeat as the defeat of a form of unruly and threatening femininity, Hodgson-Wright reads it as 'female performers whose power is epitomised by inimitable beauty' banishing 'male performers impersonating a stereotype of female transgression'.[102] This focus on beauty gets to a deeper point that with female performance – with real women's bodies taking the place of both imaginary female figures and male actors – not only is the traditional feminization of abstract virtues no longer a worn-out convention under male control, but women appear as having a unique affinity for, or privileged access to, these virtues.[103]

A song between dance sets in Jonson's *Masque of Beauty* announces:

> Had those that dwell in error foul,
> And hold that women have no soul,
> But seen these move, they would have then
> Said women were the souls of men.
> > So they do move each heart and eye
> > With the world's soul, true harmony. (307–12)

This passage cites, with exuberance, the women's dancing as incontrovertible evidence of their souls. But more than this affirmation, the provocative claim that witnesses of such a dance would conclude that 'women were the souls of men' suggests recognition of the women's agency, particularly their power to 'move' or persuade people (the word 'move' receives emphasis through repetition and metric stresses). Of course, another implication of acting as the 'souls of men' by moving them according to 'the world's soul', or 'true harmony', and indeed by correcting the view that women are soulless, is that women perform the role of a conscience. In a sense, female masquers did subtly move their audiences to address a lack of conscience in attitudes towards women and their place in political affairs, with their consistent referencing of the soul (associated with governing power and intellect) *through* the female body and not in opposition to it. An alignment of women with the soul to the disparagement or erasure of the body is as problematic

---

[101]   Ibid., 46.

[102]   Ibid., 47.

[103]   These masques' positive emphasis on beauty as synonymous with virtue counters the 'association of woman with sin through her beauty' found in 'most [Renaissance] texts' (Maclean, *Renaissance Notion of Woman*, 2.7.4). The kind of positive valuation of female beauty in the masques is perhaps similar to a neoplatonic treatment of beauty. Maclean finds that 'the most potent refutation' of the association of feminine beauty with sin occurs in 'neoplatonist writing, where the beauty of the female body is said to reflect the beauty of the soul, making beauty ... a step on the ladder to divine love'. See also Maclean, 2.11.4.

as the pervasive early modern association of women with the body. Tellingly, regarding the use of body-soul rhetoric as a tool to subordinate women, the one-sided emphasis on women's souls, and on women as having a special aptitude for virtue, instead of emphasizing the intellect, has tended to restrain women to an impossible ideal of spiritual purity and selflessness which culminates, perhaps, in the Victorian 'angel in the house' figure that Virginia Woolf so brilliantly rejects.[104] At a time when women rarely delivered lines from a formal stage, however, the masques that Queen Anna creatively influenced and participated in were not one-sided in their alignment of women with the soul. These entertainments frequently make a point about women enriching the kingdom by actively bringing a long list of gifts or virtues. The visual invocation of the soul through the female body collapses the soul-body hierarchy in a way that helps to prevent such contributions from being dismissed as either entirely bodily and so not intellectual, or as entirely spiritual or immaterial in the more negative sense of unsubstantial or inconsequential.

---

[104] Woolf, 'Professions for Women'. For an example of the problematic, unrealistic alignment of women entirely with the spiritual or the abstract, see Lisa Hopkins's reading of *The Lady's Tragedy*'s female ghost in *Female Hero*, 84–5.

Conclusion
Thomas Browne's 'great
and true *Amphibium*'[1]

Early modern understandings of the soul-body relationship, as I indicated at the beginning of this study, were multifold and complex. When soul and body were juxtaposed, however – when they were defined against each other and not in isolation – they were split along consistent gender lines. Recognizing the extent to which the body was feminized against a rational soul that was masculinized, and the role that this habitual gendering of soul and body played in naturalizing women's social and political subordination to men, is important in itself. This book has worked to demonstrate that this recognition also enables us to perceive the extent to which dramatic moments that pushed against the dominant gendered construction of soul and body in ways that involved representations of women could trouble patriarchal stereotypes and expectations by exposing their fragile roots.

And yet the selections of drama that I have explored are not primarily concerned with the soul-body dynamic. Sixteenth- and seventeenth-century texts that do explicitly address this relationship, such as devotional texts, meditations, prayers, sermons, and philosophical and theological treatises, are certainly not lacking. My focus on drama, though, reveals how the predominant gendered version of the soul-body divide – and noticeable departures from it – underwrites representations of women far beyond direct written engagement with the nature of this divide. Rosalie Osmond suggests that in drama 'one sees best the dynamic implications of the body/soul dualism worked out in its various guises', because 'conflict, essential to dramatic development, has a metaphysical foundation on which to base its human manifestations'.[2] Others, such as Lisa Hopkins, examine the representation of women's bodies or women's souls in various plays. In this study, I have sought to forward a new way of combining soul-body scholarship with theatre criticism. Instead of considering how conflict between characters might resonate with a deeper metaphysical conflict between soul and body, I have pointed to how the very structure of theatre engages the body-soul, material-immaterial dynamic. To concentrate entirely on script would seem particularly incomplete in a consideration of dramatic engagements with soul-body concepts; just as script shapes an audience's perception of the physical (recall Quarlous's

---

[1] Thomas Browne, *Religio Medici*, 39–40: 'thus is man that great and true *Amphibium*, whose nature is disposed to live not onely like other creatures in divers elements, but in divided and distinguished worlds'.

[2] Rosalie Osmond, *Mutual Accusation*, xii, see also 163.

flow of epithets for Ursula), the physical can influence our perception of the script (as when Gloriana's grin casts a critical shadow on Vindice's diatribes). In itself, this competing significance between script and material echoes and carries potential to comment on ideas of the soul-body dynamic. While we often see performance-based criticism and more traditional textual criticism to be at odds, we could not gain a sense of how the soul-body dynamic emerges onstage without considering performance alongside script. This necessity of looking at both elements at once carries implications beyond this study – what other topics become visible only when we attend to performance and text simultaneously? Finally, instead of analyzing depictions of women's bodies or souls, my study claims that creative play with the relationship between material and immaterial, spirit and body could present women in new and potentially empowering ways. This tool for subverting patriarchal gender expectations is, paradoxically, available to dramatists and perceptible to audiences because the conventional associations between masculinity and the rational soul, and femininity and the body, were so culturally engrained.

In focusing mainly on four seventeenth-century plays and a small selection of masques, my project has sampled how theatrical probing into the soul-body dynamic can translate into more positive representations of women and challenge oppressive gender ideology. My intention has not been to claim a comprehensive overview or definitive explanation of this correlation, but to demonstrate how an investigation into the impact of soul-body concepts on representations of women can open up new critical readings of plays, readings attentive to a viable, but hitherto overlooked means of questioning the patriarchal subjection of women. Through exploring tragedy, comedy, and courtly entertainment, my study shows that the relationship between depictions of women and soul-body concepts is not peculiar to a particular genre or playwright. I anticipate, rather, that the readings I have offered here suggest a new interpretive slant that is widely applicable to other early modern dramatic and non-dramatic texts.

Despite the obvious differences between the texts I selected for investigation, common themes emerged through my concentration on women and the soul-body dynamic. Puppetry was an explicit focus in the first chapter, with literal puppetry – the puppet play in *Bartholomew Fair* and Vindice's hand manipulation of Gloriana's skull in *The Revenger's Tragedy* – signalling a deeper and explicitly masculine assumption of a puppet master–like position in relation to women. Puppetry resurfaced in Chapter 2 with Maria's emphasis in *The Tamer Tamed* on maintaining her own will in order to avoid the kind of abuse that her predecessor, Kate, saw as designed to 'make a puppet' of her. Middleton revisited the macabre puppetry of *The Revenger's Tragedy* by allowing the puppeted woman a voice in *The Lady's Tragedy*, which the third chapter examined in its consideration of female ghostliness. In my final chapter I looked at how Daniel's masques for Queen Anna reframed divine possession – a form of the puppet motif – to make it an empowering as opposed to an emptying experience for women. Besides puppetry, rhetoric also ties together these plays and masques. Chapter 2's focus on Maria's strategic reversals of Petruccio's past taming techniques foregrounded rhetoric as extending to the soul-body constructs at the heart of Maria and Petruccio's conflict. In *Revenger's* rhetoric is an exercise in which Vindice can delight, but an exercise entirely at Gloriana's expense; Vindice's display of wit requires a prop and he uses his dead fiançée's skull for this purpose, setting off his intellect by debasing the material. Similarly, both Tyrant and legitimate governor rely on displays of the female body to visually mount a rhetorical justification of their position as ruler in *The Lady's Tragedy*. Dance becomes a form of rhetoric in Anna's masques, rhetoric that, like Maria's, manipulates body-soul conventions. And while dance is obviously more at issue in the masques, dance also produced significant moments in *Revenger's* and in *Tamer.* Gloriana has a revenge of sorts through the dance of death, a silent, invisible dance, but one that Vindice's staged, murderous masque dance evokes, while Maria and her army express their autonomy through mirthful dance and song. Because puppetry, rhetoric, and dance are all activities that bridge the categories of spirit and body, they are not surprising points of intersection for an investigation into the treatment of the soul-body dynamic in these very different entertainments. These intersections are of course not exhaustive, but they begin to speak to the wide variety of cultural experiences, beyond strictly religious ones, to which imaginings of the soul-body relationship are relevant.

Agreeing with Deborah Shuger that 'for exploring [dominant] culture ... it seems better not to put too much weight on theological labelling but instead to view religious discourse as a language of analysis or "ideology"',[3] I have focused throughout this project on how commonly circulating ideas about soul and body emerge in representations of women, rather than on attempting, very far, to disentangle the sometimes overlapping, sometimes conflicting nuances of specific religious orientations. These nuances, however, offer a fruitful site for future research into the interconnection between concepts of women and gendered understandings of the soul-body dynamic. Do positive views of women coincide with similar treatments of body-soul in texts with very different religious or political leanings? Or do different political and religious leanings necessitate divergent constructions of the soul-body relationship to make it compatible with more egalitarian views of women? And if religious ideas of soul and body could impact cultural views of women, could changing perspectives on and of women push back and exert pressure on religious ideas? Does a fundamental correlation exist between shifting concepts of soul and body and shifting perceptions of women?

Cultural representations of race and of class are often closely tied to treatments of gender,[4] and while these connected topics are beyond the scope of my study's

---

[3]   Deborah Kuller Shuger, *Habits of Thought*, 8.

[4]   Dympna Callaghan, *Woman and Gender in Renaissance Tragedy*, 3, goes so far as to claim that gender, as a 'category of analysis', 'can be properly understood only in juxtaposition with the analytic categories of race and class'.

initial investigation into the link between soul-body concepts and gender, further research might productively turn to the impact of these same concepts on constructions of race and class, especially since the major gendered analogy of husband and wife for the soul-body relationship was so closely associated with the political and social analogy of king and subject, lord and servant. Previous critical work has established the intersections between early modern ideas of race, class, and gender,[5] and exploring the role of soul-body ideas in these intersections would add a new dimension to this important critical work, just as it adds a new perspective to dramatic representations of women, as I have been arguing throughout this study. Above, I mention the nuances of different religious orientations as a potentially fruitful site of further study into the impact of soul-body ideas on cultural perceptions of women; specific religious nuances might also illuminate the relationship between soul-body ideas and understandings of race and class, particularly if considering politically motivated religious conversions based on changes in the official state religion, or the role religion played in transatlantic encounters.

In addition to investigating these related topics, further research into the soul-body dynamic and its shaping influence on gender ideology might produce additional questions and insights through exploring female-authored texts and non-dramatic texts. If male-authored and female-authored texts reflect shared cultural assumptions, do certain fundamental differences distinguish women's literary treatments of soul-body in relation to gender? Some of this work has already been done. Lynette McGrath, as I touched on in Chapter 2, has considered how women's writings respond to their culture's tendency to essentialize woman as body. She finds that women increasingly insist upon an 'indissoluble connection' between mind and body towards the end of the seventeenth century.[6] In her study of women philosophers in the latter half of the seventeenth century, Jacqueline Broad, too, explores women's complex views on the integration of spirit and matter. In part these views responded to Cartesian dualism, and in part they drew influence from the Cambridge School's suspicion about 'any philosophy that places a radical divide between spirit and matter', both intellectual movements that came after the period this study examines.[7] But is this later insistence, especially from women, on the indissoluble connection between spirit and matter somehow continuous with earlier theatrical representations of women that troubled the hierarchy of soul over body?

One significant difference, perhaps, between my findings and the observations of McGrath and Broad is that on the Jacobean stage, smudging the lines between spirit and matter might indeed unsettle patriarchal stereotypes about women, but it

---

[5]   See, for instance, Margo Hendricks and Patricia Parker (eds), *Women, 'Race', and Writing in the Early Modern Period*, and Mary Floyd-Wilson, *English Ethnicity and Race in Early Modern Drama*.

[6]   Lynette McGrath, *Subjectivity and Women's Poetry*, 74, n. 44.

[7]   Jacqueline Broad, *Women Philosophers*, 10–12.

can also underpin the forms of oppression that women faced. This difference makes sense in light of Shuger's assessment that, 'in the long run, the movement from premodern to modern thought describes a thickening of boundaries, but the period between 1559 and 1630 is not the long run. Rather, these years exhibit conflicting and contradictory tendencies'.[8] If boundaries were increasingly sharpening after 1630, and the solidifying line between spirit and matter perpetuated the alignment of femininity with the senses and of masculinity with 'rigorous thought',[9] opposing strict dualism would certainly be advantageous for women. But the earlier plays I have looked at tell a different story. The confusion of the boundary between spirit and matter in *Revenger's*, for instance, questions Vindice's dismissive treatment of Gloriana's skull as pure material for his use, but in *Tamer* Maria's first move in resisting Petruccio's tyranny is to force his recognition of her spirit as something separate from her body – something he cannot control through physical compulsion. The plays demonstrate that, even with the consistent gendering of spirit and matter in relation to each other, when employed as a tool to support the subordination of women, both a rigid line between soul and body (to privilege a masculinized soul as separate from and superior to a feminized body) and the collapse of this divide (to define and control women's souls through bodily surveillance and coercion) could be effective.

Even articulations of the soul-body relationship that placed soul and body on equal grounds and emphasized their mutual benefit for each other, which would seem to lend themselves to parallel articulations of gender equality – given the weight that the soul-body hierarchy has borne in upholding gender hierarchy – can be cut off from such uses. Thomas Browne's *Religio Medici*, published only a decade after the death of King James, furnishes an illustrative example. Browne views humans as 'that amphibious piece betweene a corporall and a spirituall essence, that middle frame that links those two together ... that jumps not from extreames, but unites the incompatible distances by some middle and participating natures'.[10] This view is exciting for its potential to collapse body into soul and for suggesting something about the complexity of their fusion – even, perhaps, how the 'middle frame' that a body and a soul, fused, occupy is preferable to the 'extreames' of spirit and flesh. But significantly, Browne's opinions concerning women are far less hopeful: 'man is the whole world and the breath of God' for Browne, and 'woman the rib onely and crooked piece of man'. Browne goes on to wish that humans could 'procreate like trees', without the 'triviall and vulgar' act of physical intercourse – the 'foolishest act a wise man commits in all his life'. To assure us that he has nothing against women, 'that sweet sexe', Browne explains that he is 'naturally amorous of all that is beautifull', and to prove his point, insists that he 'can looke a whole day with delight upon a handsome picture, though it be

---

[8]   Shuger, *Habits of Thought*, 11.
[9]   Broad, *Women Philosophers*.
[10] Browne, *Religio Medici*, 39.

but of an Horse'.[11] Through his association of men with 'God's breath' and women with a crooked rib and a horse, along with his regret that men are compelled to engage in such a 'foolish' physical act with women, Browne dismisses women as distinct creatures of flesh, even in the midst of articulating a vision of humans as 'amphibious', complex, in-between creatures of neither flesh nor spirit, but fully both at once.

Browne's denial, here, of the implications that this formulation of the soul-body dynamic might hold for gender relations does not mean that such implications were unavailable for appropriation. On the contrary, this book has sought to show that even when not explicitly spelled out, invocations of the spirit-matter dynamic, whether verbal or visual, inevitably impacted the way women were represented, and could open a space for positive readings of women, even in texts with misogynistic overtones like *The Revenger's Tragedy*. Browne's word 'amphibious' describes human nature at a point in between spirit and matter – not entirely one or the other. The term is also appropriate, however, to describe the versatility of the body-soul construct as a patriarchal tool of gender oppression. Jacobean dramatists, nonetheless – whether with the significant number of female audience members in mind, or perhaps as a side effect of their efforts to defend the didactic efficacy of theatre's materiality, or even quite apart from any conscious intention – represented women in ways that challenged gender hierarchy through creative re-imaginings of the soul-body construct that were equally 'amphibious'.

---

[11]   Ibid., 78.

Works Cited

Adams, Thomas. *The Workes of Tho: Adams*. London: Tho. Harper for John Grismand, 1629. STC / 948:01.

Anger, Jane. *Jane Anger Her Protection for Women*. London: Richard Jone[s] and Thomas Orwin, 1589. STC / 165:21.

Arbeau, Thoinot. *Orchesography: A Treatise in the Form of a Dialogue*. Trans. Cyril W. Beaumont. London: 1925. Rpt 1968.

Aughterson, Kate, ed. *Renaissance Woman: A Sourcebook*. London and New York: Routledge, 1995.

Axton, Marie. *The Queen's Two Bodies: Drama and the Elizabethan Succession*. London: Royal Historical Society, 1977.

Barish, Jonas. *The Antitheatrical Prejudice*. Berkeley, Los Angeles, London: U of California P, 1981.

——. '*Bartholomew Fair* and Its Puppets'. *Modern Language Quarterly* 20 (1959): 3–17.

Barroll, Leeds. *Anna of Denmark, Queen of England: A Cultural Biography*. Philadelphia: U of Pennsylvania P, 2001.

——. 'Inventing the Stuart Masque'. *The Politics of the Stuart Court Masque*. Ed. David Bevington and Peter Holbrook. Cambridge: Cambridge UP, 1998. 121–43.

Bartholomew Fair. By Ben Jonson. Dir. Antoni Cimolino. Tom Patterson Theatre, Stratford. 27 May – 2 October 2009.

Baumlin, James S. *John Donne and the Rhetorics of Renaissance Discourse*. Columbia: U of Missouri P, 1991.

Bayman, Anna and George Southcombe. 'Shrews in Pamphlets and Plays'. *Gender and Power in Shrew-Taming Narratives, 1500–1700*. Ed. David Wootton and Graham Holderness. Basingstoke: Palgrave Macmillan, 2010. 11–28.

Beaumont, Francis and John Fletcher. *The Maid's Tragedy. Four Jacobean Sex Tragedies*. Ed. Martin Wiggins. Oxford and New York: Oxford UP, 1998. 75–160.

Bedos-Rezak, Brigitte Miriam. 'Seals and Sigillography'. *Women and Gender in Medieval Europe*. Ed. Margaret Schaus. New York: Routledge, 2006. 732–3.

Bevington, David and Peter Holbrook, eds. *The Politics of the Stuart Court Masque*. Cambridge: Cambridge UP, 1998.

Bledsoe, Mary W. 'The Function of Linguistic Enormity in Ben Jonson's *Bartholomew Fair*'. *Language and Style* 17.2 (1984): 149–60.

Boose, Lynda E. '"The Getting of a Lawful Race": Racial Discourse in Early Modern England and the Unrepresentable Black Woman'. *Women, 'Race', and Writing in The Early Modern Period*. Ed. Margo Hendricks and Patricia Parker. London and New York: Routledge, 1994. 35–54.

Breton, Nicholas. *A Solemne Passion of the Soules Love*. London: George Purslowe, 1625. STC (2nd ed.) / 3698.3.

Broad, Jacqueline. *Women Philosophers of the Seventeenth Century*. Cambridge: Cambridge UP, 2002.

Brown, Pamela Allen. *Better a Shrew Than a Sheep: Women, Drama, and the Culture of Jest in Early Modern England*. Ithaca and London: Cornell UP, 2003.

Browne, Thomas. *Religio Medici and Urne-Buriall*. Ed. Stephen Greenblatt and Ramie Targoff. New York: New York Review Books, 2012.

Buccola, Regina and Lisa Hopkins, eds. *Marian Moments in Early Modern British Drama*. Aldershot: Ashgate, 2007.

Bushnell, Rebecca W. *Tragedies of Tyrants: Political Thought and Theater in the English Renaissance*. Ithaca and London: Cornell UP, 1990.

Bynum, Caroline Walker. *The Resurrection of the Body in Western Christianity, 200–1336*. New York: Columbia UP, 1995.

Callaghan, Dympna. *Woman and Gender in Renaissance Tragedy: A Study of* King Lear, Othello, The Duchess of Malfi *and* The White Devil. New York and London: Harvester Wheatsheaf, 1989.

Cartelli, Thomas. '*Bartholomew Fair* as Urban Arcadia: Jonson Responds to Shakespeare'. *Renaissance Drama* 14 (1983): 151–72.

Chapman, Alison A. 'Flaying Bartholomew: Jonson's Hagiographic Parody'. *Modern Philology* 101.4 (2004): 511–41.

Cicero. *On the Ideal Orator*. Trans. James M. May and Jakob Wisse. Oxford and New York: Oxford UP, 2001.

Clarke, Norris W. 'Living on the Edge: The Human Person as "Frontier Being" and Microcosm'. *International Philosophical Quarterly* 36.2 (1996): 183–99.

Coddon, Karin S. '"For show or useless property": Necrophilia and *The Revenger's Tragedy*'. *English Literary History* 61.1 (1994): 71–88.

Crawford, Kevin. '"All his intents are contrary to man": Softened Masculinity and Staging in Middleton's *The Lady's Tragedy*'. *Medieval and Renaissance Drama in England: An Annual Gathering of Research, Criticism and Reviews* 16 (2003): 101–29.

Cressy, David. *Birth, Marriage, and Death: Ritual, Religion, and the Life-Cycle in Tudor and Stuart England*. Oxford: Oxford UP, 1997.

Crooke, Helkiah. *Mikrokosmographia*. London: William Jaggard, 1615. STC (2nd ed.) / 6062.

Daileader, Celia. *Eroticism on the Renaissance Stage: Transcendence, Desire, and the Limits of the Visible*. Cambridge: Cambridge UP, 1998.

Daileader, Celia and Gary Taylor. Introduction. *The Tamer Tamed or, The Woman's Prize*. Ed. Celia R. Daileader and Gary Taylor. Manchester and New York: Manchester UP, 2006. 1–41.

Daniel, Samuel. *Tethys Festivall. The Order and Solemnitie of the Creation of the High and Mightie Prince Henrie*. London: John Budge, 1610. STC / 890:01.

————. *The Vision of the Twelve Goddesses. The Whole Workes of Samuel Daniel Esquire in Poetrie.* London: Nicholas Okes for Simon Waterson, 1623. STC / 1376:03.

Davies, John. *Nosce Teipsum: This Oracle Expounded in Two Elegies. 1. Of Humane Knowledge. 2. Of the Soule of Man, and the Immortalitie Thereof.* London: Richard Field for John Standish, 1599. STC (2nd ed.) / 6355.

————. 'Orchestra Or a Poeme of Dauncing'. *The Poems of Sir John Davies.* Ed. Robert Krueger. Oxford: Clarendon Press, 1975. 87–126.

Davis, Natalie Zemon. 'Women on Top'. *Feminism and Renaissance Studies.* Ed. Lorna Hutson. Oxford: Oxford UP, 1999. 156–85.

De Grazia, Margreta, Maureen Quilligan, and Peter Stallybrass, eds. *Subject and Object in Renaissance Culture.* Cambridge: Cambridge UP, 1996.

Dekker, Thomas, John Ford, and William Rowley. *The Witch of Edmonton.* Ed. Peter Corbin and Douglas Sedge. Manchester and New York: Manchester UP, 1999.

Diehl, Huston. *Staging Reform, Reforming the Stage: Protestantism and Popular Theater in Early Modern England.* Ithaca: Cornell UP, 1997.

DiPasquale, Theresa M. *Refiguring the Sacred Feminine: The Poems of John Donne, Aemilia Lanyer, and John Milton.* Pittsburgh: Duquesne UP, 2008.

Dolan, Frances. 'Hermione's Ghost: Catholicism, the Feminine, and the Undead'. *The Impact of Feminism in English Renaissance Studies.* Ed. Dympna Callaghan. Basingstoke: Palgrave Macmillan, 2007.

Dollimore, Jonathan. *Radical Tragedy: Religion, Ideology and Power in the Drama of Shakespeare and His Contemporaries.* Brighton, Sussex: The Harvester Press, 1984.

Donne, John. 'To Sir [Henry Goodyer]'. *The Complete Poetry and Selected Prose of John Donne.* Ed. Charles M. Coffin. New York: Modern Library, 2001. 383–4.

————. 'A Valediction: Forbidding Mourning'. *The Complete Poetry and Selected Prose of John Donne.* Ed. Charles M. Coffin. New York: Modern Library, 2001. 38–9.

————. 'Why Hath the Common Opinion Affoorded Woemen Soules?' *Paradoxes and Problems.* Ed. Helen Peters. Oxford: Clarendon; New York: Oxford UP, 1980.

Dunn-Hensley, Susan. 'Whore Queens: The Sexualized Female Body and the State'. *'High and Mighty Queens' of Early Modern England: Realities and Representations.* Ed. Carole Levin et al. New York: Palgrave Macmillan, 2003. 101–16.

Eaton, Sara. '"Content with art"?: Seeing the Emblematic Woman in *The Second Maiden's Tragedy* and *The Winter's Tale*'. *Shakespearean Power and Punishment: A Volume of Essays.* Ed. Gillian Murray Kendall. Madison, NJ and London, England: Fairleigh Dickinson UP, 1998. 59–86.

Egan, Gabriel. 'The Use of Booths in the Original Staging of Jonson's *Bartholomew Fair*'. *Cahiers Élisabéthains* 53 (1998): 43–52.

Eggert, Katherine. *Showing Like a Queen: Female Authority and Literary Experiment in Spenser, Shakespeare, and Milton*. Philadelphia: U of Pennsylvania P, 2000.

Elyot, Thomas. *The Boke Named the Governour*. London: Tho. Bertheleti, 1531. STC / 35:01.

Farlie, Robert. *Lychnocausia*. London: Tho. Cotes for Michael Sparke Junior, 1638. STC / 790:15.

Fernie, Ewan, Ramona Wray, et al., eds. *Reconceiving the Renaissance: A Critical Reader*. Oxford: Oxford UP, 2005.

Findlay, Alison. *A Feminist Perspective on Renaissance Drama*. Oxford: Blackwell, 1999.

Finin, Kathryn R. '"Wild Justice" and the Female Body in *The Revenger's Tragedy*'. *Renaissance Forum* 6.2 (2003): 22 par.

Fletcher, Anthony. *Gender, Sex and Subordination in England 1500–1800*. New Haven and London: Yale UP, 1995.

Fletcher, John. *The Noble Gentleman. The Dramatic Works in The Beaumont and Fletcher Canon*. Vol. 3. Ed. Fredson Bowers. Cambridge: Cambridge UP, 1976. 113–224.

———. *The Tamer Tamed or, The Woman's Prize*. Ed. Celia R. Daileader and Gary Taylor. Manchester and New York: Manchester UP, 2006.

Floyd-Wilson, Mary. *English Ethnicity and Race in Early Modern Drama*. Cambridge: Cambridge UP, 2003.

Folkerth, Wes. *The Sound of Shakespeare*. London and New York: Routledge, 2002.

Freud, Sigmund. 'The Uncanny'. *Literary Theory: An Anthology*. 2nd ed. Ed. Julie Rivkin and Michael Ryan. Malden, MA: Blackwell, 1998. Rpt 2004. 418–30.

Gascoigne, George. 'The Steele Glas'. *English Sixteenth-Century Verse: An Anthology*. Ed. Richard S. Sylvester. New York and London: Norton, 1974. Rpt 1984. 275–316.

Gittings, Clare. *Death, Burial, and the Individual in Early Modern England*. London and Sydney: Croom Helm, 1984.

Goldberg, Jonathan. *James I and the Politics of Literature*. Stanford: Stanford UP, 1983.

———, ed. *Queering the Renaissance*. Durham and London: Duke UP, 1994.

Gough, Melinda. 'Jonson's Siren Stage'. *Studies in Philology* 96.1 (1999): 68–95.

Gowing, Laura. *Domestic Dangers: Women, Words, and Sex in Early Modern London*. Oxford: Clarendon; Oxford and Toronto: Oxford UP, 1996.

———. 'Gender and the Language of Insult in Early Modern London'. *History Workshop Journal* 35 (1993): 1–21.

Grant, Patrick. *Literature and the Discovery of Method in the English Renaissance*. London: Macmillan, 1985.

Greene, Thomas M. 'Ben Jonson and the Centered Self'. *Studies in English Literature* 10.2 (1970): 325–48.

Gundersheimer, Werner L. Introduction. *The Dance of Death by Hans Holbein the Younger: A Complete Facsimile of the Original 1538 Edition of Les Simulachres & historiees faces de la mort.* New York: Dover, 1971. i–xiv.

Hanson, Elizabeth. *Discovering the Subject in Renaissance England.* Cambridge: Cambridge UP, 1998.

Harp, Richard. 'Catholicism'. 'Jonson and his Era: Overviews of Modern Research'. *Ben Jonson Journal* 14.1 (2007): 112–16.

Harward, Simon. *A Discourse Concerning the Soule and Spirit of Man.* London: John Windet, 1604. STC (2nd ed.) / 12917.

Haslem, Lori Schroeder. '"Troubled with the Mother": Longings, Purgings, and the Maternal Body in *Bartholomew Fair* and *The Duchess of Malfi'. Modern Philology* 92.4 (1995): 438–60.

Haynes, Jonathan. *The Social Relations of Jonson's Theater.* Cambridge: Cambridge UP, 1992.

Hendricks, Margo and Patricia Parker, eds. *Women, 'Race', and Writing in The Early Modern Period.* London and New York: Routledge, 1994.

Herbert, George. 'Church-Monuments'. *George Herbert: The Complete English Poems.* Ed. John Tobin. London: Penguin, 1991. Rpt 2004.

Herford, Percy C.H. and Evelyn Simpson. *Ben Jonson.* Vol. X. Oxford: Clarendon, 1950.

Hill, William. *The Infancie of the Soule; or, The Soule of an Infant.* London: W. W[hite] for C. Knight, 1605. STC (2nd ed.) / 13506.

Hodgson, Elizabeth M.A. *Gender and the Sacred Self in John Donne.* Newark: U of Delaware P; London: Associated UP, 1999.

Hodgson-Wright, Stephanie. 'Beauty, Chastity and Wit: Feminising the Centre-Stage'. *Women and Dramatic Production 1550–1700.* Ed. Alison Findlay and Stephanie Hodgson-Wright. Harlow, England and New York: Longman, 2000. 42–67.

Holbein, Hans. *The Dance of Death by Hans Holbein the Younger: A Complete Facsimile of the Original 1538 Edition of Les Simulachres & historiees faces de la mort.* New York: Dover, 1971.

Holbrook, Peter. 'Jacobean Masques and the Jacobean Peace'. *The Politics of the Stuart Court Masque.* Ed. David Bevington and Peter Holbrook. Cambridge: Cambridge UP, 1998. 67–87.

Hopkins, Lisa. *The Female Hero in Renaissance Tragedy.* Basingstoke, Hampshire and New York: Palgrave Macmillan, 2002.

Howard, Skiles. *The Politics of Courtly Dancing in Early Modern England.* Amherst: U of Massachusetts P, 1998.

James I. *Basilikon Doron, Or, His Maiesties Instructions to His Dearest Sonne, Henry the Prince.* Edinburgh: Felix Kyngston for John Norton, 1603. STC / 993:12.

Jankowski, Theodora A. *Women in Power in the Early Modern Drama.* Urbana and Chicago: U of Illinois P, 1992.

Jensen, Ejner J. *Ben Jonson's Comedies on the Modern Stage*. Ann Arbor: UMI Research P, 1985.

Jones, Ann Rosalind and Peter Stallybrass. *Renaissance Clothing and the Materials of Memory*. Cambridge and New York: Cambridge UP, 2000.

Jonson, Ben. *Bartholomew Fair*. *Jonson: Four Comedies*. Ed. Helen Ostovich. London and New York: Longman, 1997. 541–688.

———. 'Epigram LXXVI: On Lucy, Countess of Bedford'. *The New Oxford Book of Seventeenth-Century Verse*. Ed. Alastair Fowler. Oxford: Oxford UP, 1991. Rpt 2002. 128.

———. *Every Man Out of His Humour*. Ed. Helen Ostovich. Manchester and New York: Manchester UP; New York: Palgrave, 2001.

———. *Hymenaei, or the Solemnities of Masque and Barriers at a Marriage. Ben Jonson: The Complete Masques*. Ed. Stephen Orgel. New Haven and London: Yale UP, 1969. Rpt 1975. 75–106.

———. *Love's Triumph Through Callipolis. Ben Jonson: The Complete Masques*. Ed. Stephen Orgel. New Haven and London: Yale UP, 1969. Rpt 1975. 454–61.

———. *The Masque of Beauty. Ben Jonson: The Complete Masques*. Ed. Stephen Orgel. New Haven and London: Yale UP, 1969. Rpt 1975. 61–74.

———. *The Masque of Blackness. Masques of Difference: Four Court Masques by Ben Jonson*. Ed. Kristen McDermott. Manchester and New York: Manchester UP, 2007. 91–105.

———. *The Masque of Queens. Masques of Difference: Four Court Masques by Ben Jonson*. Ed. Kristen McDermott. Manchester and New York: Manchester UP, 2007. 106–32.

———. *Timber or Discoveries*. Ed. Ralph S. Walker. Syracuse UP, 1953.

Karim-Cooper, Farah. *Cosmetics in Shakespearean and Renaissance Drama*. Edinburgh: Edinburgh UP, 2006.

Kay, David W. *Ben Jonson: A Literary Life*. London: Macmillan, 1995.

Keller, Eve. *Generating Bodies and Gendered Selves: The Rhetoric of Reproduction in Early Modern England*. Seattle and London: U of Washington P, 2007.

Kelly, Kathleen Coyne and Marina Leslie, eds. *Menacing Virgins: Representing Virginity in the Middle Ages and Renaissance*. Newark: U of Delaware P, 1999.

Kennedy, Gwynne. *Just Anger: Representing Women's Anger in Early Modern England*. Carbondale and Edwardsville: Southern Illinois UP, 2000.

Kiening, Christian. 'Le Double décomposé: rencontres des vivants et des morts à la fin du Moyen Age'. *Annales* 50.5 (1995): 1157–90.

King James Bible. London: Robert Barker, 1611; Cambridge: Chadwyck-Healey, 1996.

Knox, John. *The First Blast of the Trumpet Against the Monstrous Regiment of Women*. London, 1558. STC / 253:09.

Kurtz, Léonard P. *The Dance of Death and the Macabre Spirit in European Literature*. New York: 1934. Rpt Geneva: Slatkine, 1975.

Lada-Richards, I. '"In the Mirror of the Dance": A Lucianic Metaphor in Its Performative and Ethical Contexts'. *Mnemosyne*, 4th series, 58.3 (2005): 335–57.

Lancashire, Anne Begor, ed. *The Second Maiden's Tragedy*. Manchester: Manchester UP, 1978.

Lancashire, Ian, ed. *Lexicons of Early Modern English*. U of Toronto P, 2013.

Langley, Eric F. 'Anatomizing the Early-Modern Eye: A Literary Case Study'. *Renaissance Studies* 20.3 (2006): 340–55.

Lanyer, Aemilia. *The Poems of Aemilia Lanyer: Salve Deus Rex Judaeorum*. Ed. Susanne Woods. New York and Oxford: Oxford UP, 1993.

Laqueur, Thomas. *Making Sex: Body and Gender from the Greeks to Freud*. Cambridge, MA and London: Harvard UP, 1990.

Leggatt, Alexander. *Introduction to English Renaissance Comedy*. Manchester and New York: Manchester UP, 1999.

Levin, Carole. *'The Heart and Stomach of a King': Elizabeth I and the Politics of Sex and Power*. Philadelphia: U of Pennsylvania P, 1994.

Levin, Richard. 'The Double Plot of *The Second Maiden's Tragedy*'. *Studies in English Literature 1500–1900* 3.2 (1963): 219–31.

Lewalski, Barbara Kiefer. *Writing Women in Jacobean England*. Cambridge, MA: Harvard UP, 1993.

Liebler, Naomi Conn, ed. *The Female Tragic Hero in English Renaissance Drama*. New York: Palgrave, 2002.

Limon, Jerzy. *The Masque of Stuart Culture*. Newark: U of Delaware P; London and Toronto: Associated UP, 1990.

Lloyd, Genevieve. *The Man of Reason: 'Male' and 'Female' in Western Philosophy*. 2nd ed. Minneapolis: U of Minnesota P, 1993.

Lodhia, Sheetal. '"The house is hers, the soul is but a tenant": Material Self-Fashioning and Revenge Tragedy.' *Early Theatre* 12.2 (2009): 135–61.

Longfellow, Erica. *Women and Religious Writing in Early Modern England*. Cambridge and New York: Cambridge UP, 2004.

Loughlin, Marie H. *Hymeneutics: Interpreting Virginity on the Early Modern Stage*. Lewisburg: Bucknell UP; London and Cranbury, NJ: Associated UP, 1997.

Mackay, Ellen. *Persecution, Plague, and Fire: Fugitive Histories of the Stage in Early Modern England*. Chicago: U of Chicago P, 2011.

Maclean, Ian. 'The Notion of Woman in Medicine, Anatomy, and Physiology'. *Feminism and Renaissance Studies*. Ed. Lorna Hutson. Oxford: Oxford UP, 1999. 127–55.

————. *The Renaissance Notion of Woman: A Study in the Fortunes of Scholasticism and Medical Science in European Intellectual Life*. Cambridge: Cambridge UP, 1980. Rpt 1985, 1987.

Manning, Roger B. *Village Revolts: Social Protest and Popular Disturbances in England, 1509–1640*. Oxford: Clarendon; New York: Oxford UP, 1988.

Marcus, Leah S. *The Politics of Mirth: Jonson, Herrick, Milton, Marvell, and the Defense of Old Holiday Pastimes*. Chicago and London: U of Chicago P, 1986.

Marston, John. *Sophonisba. The Malcontent and Other Plays*. Ed. Keith Sturgess. Oxford: Oxford UP, 1997. 241–94.

Martin, Mathew R. *Between Theater and Philosophy: Skepticism in the Major City Comedies of Ben Jonson and Thomas Middleton*. Newark: U of Delaware P; London: Associated UP, 2001.

Martin, Paul. 'The Body in the Realm of Desire: Gendered Images on the Horizon of the Divine'. *Mystics Quarterly* 30.3–4 (2004): 96–121.

Massinger, Philip. *The Duke of Milan. The Selected Plays of Philip Massinger*. Ed. Colin Gibson. Cambridge: Cambridge UP, 1978. 7–93.

Maurer, Margaret. 'Constering Bianca: *The Taming of the Shrew* and *The Woman's Prize, or The Tamer Tamed*'. *Medieval and Renaissance Drama in England* 14 (2001): 186–206.

Maus, Katharine Eisaman. *Inwardness and Theatre in the English Renaissance*. Chicago and London: U of Chicago P, 1995.

McAdam, Ian. 'The Puritan Dialectic of Law and Grace in *Bartholomew Fair*'. *Studies in English Literature 1500–1900* 46.2 (2006): 415–33.

McGrath, Lynette. 'The Other Body: Women's Inscription of Their Physical Images in 16th- and 17th-Century England'. *Women's Studies* 26.1 (1997): 27–58.

———. *Subjectivity and Women's Poetry in Early Modern England: 'Why on the ridge should she desire to go?'* Aldershot: Ashgate, 2002.

McManus, Clare. 'Memorialising Anna of Denmark's Court'. *Women and Culture at the Courts of the Stuart Queens*. Ed. Clare McManus. Houndmills, Basingstoke, Hampshire, and New York: 2003. 81–99.

———. *Women on the Renaissance Stage: Anna of Denmark and Female Masquing in the Stuart Court (1590–1619)*. Manchester and New York: Manchester UP, 2002.

McMullan, Gordon. *The Politics of Unease in the Plays of John Fletcher*. Amherst: U of Massachusetts P, 1994.

McNeill, Fiona. 'Gynocentric London Spaces: (Re)Locating Masterless Women in Early Stuart Drama'. *Renaissance Drama* 28 (1997): 195–244.

Mendelson, Sara and Patricia Crawford. *Women in Early Modern England 1550–1720*. Oxford: Clarendon, 1998.

Middleton, Thomas. *The Lady's Tragedy. The Collected Works of Thomas Middleton*. Ed. Gary Taylor and John Lavagnino. Oxford: Clarendon, 2007. 833–906.

———. *The Revenger's Tragedy* (New Mermaids). Ed. Brian Gibbons. New York: Norton, 1991.

Middleton, Thomas and William Rowley. *The Changeling. The Collected Works of Thomas Middleton.* Ed. Gary Taylor and John Lavagnino. Oxford: Clarendon, 2007. 1632–78.

Milton, John. *A Masque ... Presented at Ludlow Castle. John Milton: The Major Works*. Ed. Stephen Orgel and Jonathan Goldberg. Oxford: Oxford UP, 1991. 44–71.

———. *Paradise Lost*. 2nd ed. Ed. Scott Elledge. New York and London: Norton, 1993.

Mirabella, M. Bella. 'Mute Rhetorics: Women, the Gaze, and Dance in Renaissance England'. *Genre* 28 (1995): 413–44.

Morford, Mark P.O. and Robert J. Lenardon. *Classical Mythology*. 7th ed. New York and Oxford: Oxford UP, 2003.

Mullaney, Steven. 'Mourning and Misogyny: *Hamlet, The Revenger's Tragedy*, and the Final Progress of Elizabeth I, 1600–1607'. *Centuries' Ends, Narrative Means*. Ed. Robert Newman. Stanford: Stanford UP, 1996. 240–60.

Narveson, Kate. 'Flesh, Excrement, Humors, Nothing: The Body in Early Stuart Devotional Discourse'. *Studies in Philology* 96.3 (1999): 313–33.

Nelson, Victoria. *The Secret Life of Puppets*. Cambridge, MA and London: Harvard UP, 2001.

O'Callaghan, Michelle. 'Dreaming the Dead: Ghosts and History in the Early Seventeenth Century'. *Reading the Early Modern Dream: The Terrors of the Night*. Ed. Katharine Hodgkin et al. New York: Routledge, 2008. 81–96.

O'Malley, Susan Gushee, ed. *Defences of Women: Jane Anger, Rachel Speght, Ester Sowernam, and Constantia Munda*. Aldershot, England: Scholar; Brookfield, VT: Ashgate, 1996.

Oosterwijk, Sophie. 'Of Corpses, Constables, and Kings: The Danse Macabre in Late Medieval and Renaissance Culture'. *Journal of the British Archaeological Association* 157 (2004): 61–90.

Orgel, Stephen. *The Illusion of Power: Political Theater in the English Renaissance*. Berkeley, Los Angeles, and London: U of California P, 1975.

——. *Impersonations: The Performance of Gender in Shakespeare's England*. Cambridge: Cambridge UP, 1996.

——. 'Marginal Jonson'. *The Politics of the Stuart Court Masque*. Ed. David Bevington and Peter Holbrook. Cambridge: Cambridge UP, 1998. 144–75.

Osmond, Rosalie. *Imagining the Soul: A History*. Stroud: Sutton, 2003.

——. *Mutual Accusation: Seventeenth-Century Body and Soul Dialogues in Their Literary and Theological Context*. Toronto, Buffalo, and London: U of Toronto P, 1990.

Oxford English Dictionary. OED Online. Oxford UP. http://www.oed.com.

Palmer, Barbara D. 'Staging Invisibility in English Early Modern Drama'. *Early Theatre* 11.2 (2008): 113–28.

Parfitt, George A.E. *John Donne: A Literary Life*. New York: St. Martin's, 1989.

Parker, Patricia. 'Literary Fat Ladies and the Generation of the Text'. *Feminism and Renaissance Studies*. Ed. Lorna Hutson. Oxford: Oxford UP, 1999. 249–85.

——. *Literary Fat Ladies: Rhetoric, Gender, Property*. London and New York: Methuen, 1987.

Paster, Gail Kern. *The Body Embarrassed: Drama and the Disciplines of Shame in Early Modern England*. Ithaca: Cornell UP, 1993.

——. 'Nervous Tension: Networks of Blood and Spirit in the Early Modern Body'. *The Body in Parts: Fantasies of Corporeality in Early Modern Europe*. Ed. David Hillman and Carla Mazzio. New York: Routledge, 1997. 107–25.

Perfetti, Lisa, ed. *The Representation of Women's Emotions in Medieval and Early Modern Culture*. Gainesville: UP of Florida, 2005.

Peters, Helen, ed. *Paradoxes and Problems*. Oxford: Clarendon; New York: Oxford UP, 1980.

Pinciss, G.M. '*Bartholomew Fair* and Jonsonian Tolerance'. *Studies in English Literature 1500–1900* 35.2 (1995): 345–59.

Pollard, Tanya. *Drugs and Theatre in Early Modern England*. Oxford: Oxford UP, 2005.

Pope, Johnathan. 'An Anatomy of the Soul in English Renaissance Religious Poetry'. Diss., McMaster University, 2009.

Quarles, Francis. *Emblemes*. London: G.M. for John Marriot, 1635. STC / 904:03 and STC / 1779:28.

———. *Hieroglyphikes of the Life of Man*. London: M. Flesher for John Marriot, 1638. STC / 934:02.

Ravelhofer, Barbara. *The Early Stuart Masque: Dance, Costume, Music*. Oxford: Oxford UP, 2006.

Ray, Robert H. *A John Donne Companion*. New York: Garland, 1990.

Rebhorn, Wayne A. *The Emperor of Men's Minds: Literature and the Renaissance Discourse of Rhetoric*. Ithaca and London: Cornell UP, 1995.

Rhodes, Neil. *Elizabethan Grotesque*. London: Routledge, 1980.

———. *The Power of Eloquence and English Renaissance Literature*. New York: St. Martin's, 1992.

Richards, Jennifer and Alison Thorne, eds. *Rhetoric, Women, and Politics in Early Modern England*. London: Routledge, 2006.

Richardson, Ruth. *Death, Dissection and the Destitute*. 2nd ed. Chicago and London: U of Chicago P, 1987, 2000.

Rist, Thomas. *Revenge Tragedy and the Drama of Commemoration in Reforming England*. Aldershot: Ashgate, 2008.

Savage, James E. *Ben Jonson's Basic Comic Characters and Other Essays*. Mississippi: University and College P of Mississippi, 1973.

Schafer, Elizabeth. *Ms-Directing Shakespeare: Women Direct Shakespeare*. New York: St. Martin's, 2000.

Schoenfeldt, Michael. *Bodies and Selves in Early Modern England: Physiology and Inwardness in Spenser, Shakespeare, Herbert, and Milton*. Cambridge: Cambridge UP, 1999.

Shakespeare, William. *Cymbeline. The Complete Works of Shakespeare*. 5th ed. Ed. David Bevington. New York: Pearson Longman, 2004. 1475–526.

———. *The First Part of King Henry the Fourth. The Complete Works of Shakespeare*. 5th ed. Ed. David Bevington. New York: Pearson Longman, 2004. 784–825.

———. *Hamlet, Prince of Denmark. The Complete Works of Shakespeare*. 5th ed. Ed. David Bevington. New York: Pearson Longman, 2004. 1091–149.

———. *A Midsummer Night's Dream. The Complete Works of Shakespeare*. 5th ed. Ed. David Bevington. New York: Pearson Longman, 2004. 148–79.

———. *Othello, the Moor of Venice. The Complete Works of Shakespeare*. 5th ed. Ed. David Bevington. New York: Pearson Longman, 2004. 1150–200.

————. *The Rape of Lucrece. The Complete Works of Shakespeare.* 5th ed. Ed. David Bevington. New York: Pearson Longman, 2004. 1674–97.

————. *The Taming of the Shrew. The Complete Works of Shakespeare.* 5th ed. Ed. David Bevington. New York: Pearson Longman, 2004. 108–47.

————. *The Tempest. The Complete Works of Shakespeare.* 5th ed. Ed. David Bevington. New York: Pearson Longman, 2004. 1570–603.

————. *The Winter's Tale. The Complete Works of Shakespeare.* 5th ed. Ed. David Bevington. New York: Pearson Longman, 2004. 1527–69.

Sharpe, Kevin. *Selling the Tudor Monarchy: Authority and Image in Sixteenth-Century England.* New Haven and London: Yale UP, 2009.

Shershow, Scott Cutler. *Puppets and 'Popular' Culture.* Ithaca and London: Cornell UP, 1995.

Shuger, Debora Kuller. *Habits of Thought in the English Renaissance: Religion, Politics, and the Dominant Culture.* Toronto, Buffalo, and London: U of Toronto P, 1997.

————. 'Hypocrites and Puppets in *Bartholomew Fair'. Modern Philology* 82.1 (1984): 70–73.

Sidney, Philip. *A Defence of Poetry.* Ed. J.A. Van Dorsten. Oxford: Oxford UP, 1966.

Simpson, Evelyn. *A Study of the Prose Works of John Donne.* Oxford: Clarendon, 1948.

Sloan, Larue Love. '"Caparisoned like the horse": Tongue and Tail in Shakespeare's *The Taming of the Shrew'. Early Modern Literary Studies* 10.2 (2004). 1.1–24.

Smith, Molly Easo. 'John Fletcher's Response to the Gender Debate: *The Woman's Prize* and *The Taming of the Shrew'. Papers on Language and Literature* 31.1 (1995): 38–60.

Speaight, George. *The History of the English Puppet Theatre.* London, Toronto, Wellington, and Sydney: George G. Harrap & Co., 1955.

Spenser, Edmund. *The Faerie Queene. Edmund Spenser's Poetry.* 3rd ed. Ed. Hugh Maclean and Anne Lake Prescott. New York: Norton, 1993.

Stallybrass, Peter. 'Hauntings: The Materiality of Memory on the Renaissance Stage'. *Generation and Degeneration: Tropes of Reproduction in Literature and History from Antiquity through Early Modern Europe.* Ed. Valeria Finucci and Kevin Brownlee. Durham, NC: Duke UP, 2001. 287–316.

————. 'Reading the Body: *The Revenger's Tragedy* and the Jacobean Theater of Consumption'. *Renaissance Drama* 18 (1987): 121–41.

Sullivan, Mary. *Court Masques of James I: Their Influence on Shakespeare and the Public Theatres.* New York: Russell and Russell, 1913. Rpt 1973.

The Taming of the Tamer. By John Fletcher. Dir. Patrick Young. Theatre Erindale, Mississauga. 24 March 2009.

Thomas, Keith. *Religion and the Decline of Magic: Studies in Popular Beliefs in Sixteenth and Seventeenth Century England.* London: Weidenfeld and Nicolson, 1971.

Tomlinson, Sophie. *Women on Stage in Stuart Drama.* Cambridge: Cambridge UP, 2005.

Vickers, Brian. *In Defence of Rhetoric*. Oxford: Clarendon, 1988.

Walker, Julia M. 'Bones of Contention: Posthumous Images of Elizabeth and Stuart Politics'. *Dissing Elizabeth: Negative Representations of Gloriana*. Ed. Julia M. Walker. Durham and London: Duke UP, 1998.

Wall, Wendy. *The Imprint of Gender: Authorship and Publication in the English Renaissance*. Ithaca and London: Cornell UP, 1993.

Walter, Melissa. 'Dramatic Bodies and Novellesque Spaces in Jacobean Tragedy'. *Transnational Exchange in Early Modern Theater*. Ed. Robert Henke and Eric Nicholson. Aldershot: Ashgate, 2008. 63–77.

Watson, Robert N. *Ben Jonson's Parodic Strategy: Literary Imperialism in the Comedies*. Cambridge, MA: Harvard UP, 1987.

Wayne, Valerie. 'The Dearth of the Author: Anonymity's Allies and *Swetname the Woman-Hater*'. Ed. Susan Frye and Karen Robertson. *Maids and Mistresses, Cousins and Queens: Women's Alliances in Early Modern England*. Oxford: Oxford UP, 1999. 221–40.

Webster, John. *The Duchess of Malfi*. Ed. Leah S. Marcus. London: Arden Shakespeare, 2009.

Woolf, Virginia. 'Professions for Women'. *The Norton Anthology of English Literature*. 7th ed. Vol. 2. Ed. M.H. Abrams et al. New York and London: Norton, 2000. 2214–18.

Woolnor, Henry. *The True Originall of the Soule*. London: T. Paine and M. Symmons, 1641. Wing / W3526.

Woolton, John. *A Treatise of the Immortalitie of the Soule wherein is declared the origine, nature, and powers of the same*. London: [Thomas Purfoote for] John Shepperd, 1576. STC (2nd ed.) / 25979.

Wootton, David. '*The Tamer Tamed*, or None Shall Have Prizes: "Equality" in Shakespeare's England'. *Gender and Power in Shrew-Taming Narratives, 1500–1700*. Ed. David Wootton and Graham Holderness. Basingstoke: Palgrave Macmillan, 2010. 206–25.

Wootton, David and Graham Holderness, eds. *Gender and Power in Shrew-Taming Narratives, 1500–1700*. Basingstoke: Palgrave Macmillan, 2010.

Wright, John P. and Paul Potter, eds. *Psyche and Soma: Physicians and Metaphysicians on the Mind-Body Problem from Antiquity to Enlightenment*. Oxford: Oxford UP, 2000.

Wright, Thomas. *The Passions of the Minde in Generall*. London: Valentine Simmes [and Adam Islip] for Walter Burre [and Thomas Thorpe], 1604. STC (2nd ed.) / 26040.

Zimmerman, Susan. *The Early Modern Corpse and Shakespeare's Theatre*. Edinburgh: Edinburgh UP, 2005.

———. 'Marginal Man: The Representation of Horror in Renaissance Tragedy'. *Discontinuities: New Essays on Renaissance Literature and Criticism*. Ed. Viviana Comensoli and Paul Stevens. Toronto: U of Toronto P, 1998. 159–78.

Index